Toward Painless Writing: A Guide for Health Professionals

Tova Navarra, BA, RN

SLACK Incorporated, 6900 Grove Road, Thorofare, NJ 08086

Publisher: John H. Bond
Editorial Director: Amy E. Drummond
Creative Director: Linda Baker
Assistant Editor: Elisabeth DeBoer
Copyright © 1998 by SLACK Incorporated

Navarra, Tova.
    Toward painless writing: a guide for health
professionals/Tova Navarra.
        p. cm.
    Includes bibliographical references and index.
    ISBN 1-55642-293-8
    1. Medical writing—Handbooks, manuals, etc.   I. Title
R119.N38   1998
808'.06661—dc21   98-12762
                                  CIP

Printed in the United States of America

Published by: SLACK Incorporated
                  6900 Grove Road
                  Thorofare, NJ 08086 USA
                  Telephone: 609-848-1000
                  Fax: 609-853-5991
                  Website: www.slackinc.com

Last digit is print number: 10 9 8 7 6 5 4 3 2 1

Dedication

I dedicate this book to my daughter, Yolanda,
who wears many hats with sweetness and aplomb:
journalist, creative writer, certified massage therapist,
musician, artist, and healer.
God go with you everywhere, my little lamb.

And to her husband, Guy Fleming, with love and hope for
his happiness, and the realization of his many talents.

And to my step-grandchildren, Amanda and Wesley
Fleming, who are adorable and fun, and who remind me
that love and laughter are what makes life worth living.

Contents

Writing for Your Professional Life
Take Mental Notes on Everything
Respect the Written Language
The Authoritative Look of Print
Writing Is as Easy as Bleeding
Use Your Imagination Even in Academic and
    Nonfiction Writing
No Time to Write?
Products of Passion
Reassurance Is Always Welcome
Teach Unabashedly
Start With a Loving Desire to Write
Use a Computer, Typewriter, or Pen, as Long as
    You Use Your Ability to Write
Confidentiality in Health Care Writing
If You Can Say It, You Can Write It
Hearing What You Write
Reading Teaches You to Write
So What if Your Name Isn't Hemingway?
You Don't Need to Put on Airs in Writing
Be Open to Your Accumulated Experience
    as a Caregiver

Write What You Know
Write a First Sentence That Compels the Reader
    to Read On

Acknowledgments

Thank you, thank you, all you dear ones who inspire and encourage me, particularly:

- John Bond, Publisher, and Amy Drummond, Editorial Director, both of SLACK Incorporated, who asked me to write this book and graciously provided helpful materials I would not have come across on my own.

- Margaret Lundrigan, MSW, co-author and friend-to-the-end, who daily listens to my writhings and offers therapy that would otherwise cost me my life savings.

- Author extraordinaire Anne Lamott, whose book *Bird by Bird: Some Instructions on Writing and Life* strengthened my will to write, to accept myself as a writer (good, bad, or mediocre), and to complete this book with a heart that is grateful I made it through nursing school so I can also participate in one of the most mysterious and powerful industries on Earth—health care.

- Louis de Furia, former publisher of *New Jersey Music & Arts Magazine*, the late Helen Aumack of the Community Relations department of Jersey Shore Medical Center, and other writers and editors who taught me about clear, honest writing.

- My son, Johnny, who writes strange and beautiful songs, stories, and poems, and my beloved shih tzu, Francis, who stays at my feet for hours as I type.

About the Author

Tova Navarra is a magna cum laude graduate of Seton Hall University, a registered nurse, former contributing editor of the *American Journal of Nursing* and syndicated health columnist for Copley News Service, and the author of 14 diverse books. Her books include: *Images of America: Staten Island*; *Images of America: Levittown—The First Fifty Years; Images of America: Howell and Farmingdale—A Social and Cultural History; Wisdom for Caregivers; An Insider's Guide to Home Health Care; On My Own: Helping Kids Help Themselves; Therapeutic Communication; Allergies A-Z; The Encyclopedia of Vitamins, Minerals, and Supplements; Your Body: Highlights of Human Anatomy; The New Jersey Shore: A Vanishing Splendor*, a novel, a volume of poems, and two plays. Also a former feature writer and art critic for the *Asbury Park Press* and the mother of two grown children, Ms. Navarra is working on several new books for both adults and children. She is also certified in Therapeutic Touch and studying to become a Reiki master. Ms. Navarra is listed in *Who's Who in American Nursing* and *Who's Who of American Women (1997-1998, 20th ed)*. She lives in Monmouth County, New Jersey.

Prologue

When I was an opinionated child shooting my mouth off, my father would roar, "**You have nothing to say!**"

Because of that exclamation, which to this day echoes in my mind, two things concurrently happened to me: I suffer feeling stupid and unworthy, and I get a big kick out of the fact that I became a writer anyway.

I never stop admiring great writers and never stop aspiring to be one. I keep in mind Jack Kerouac's intimidating words: "Walking on water wasn't built in a day."

Preface

Author Lewis Carroll, best known for *Alice's Adventures in Wonderland*, referred to reading and writing as "reeling and writhing." Unfortunately, the two activities can be as painful as Carroll described, especially "writhing," which is why I am writing this book—for you, of course, who seek relief from pain attributable to writing anything from an incident report to a doctoral dissertation —and for me. Authors ought to have a little fun, after all, and I think most of the time I do. I hope this book helps adjust your attitude, the main cause of distress, toward writing. I believe many people grow a tumor at the thought of writing, so it has been given a bad rap from the outset. But writing need not require a morphine drip. Essentially, it requires a light heart, the proper tricks of the trade, and a "just do it" approach.

Television story editor Lawrence G. DiTillio wrote an article for the February 1997 issue of *Writer's Digest* that doled out a hefty measure of help for those interested in TV scriptwriting. One of the strongest tips he offered was to take a journalistic approach, i.e., follow the five Ws: who, what, when, where, and why. DiTillio supports my sentiments exactly, whether you are writing a book report, an article for a professional journal, a therapeutic drama for role-playing, a book on diet and exercise, or a letter to your mother. If whatever you write does not contain all five Ws, which amount to questions you need to answer for your readers, something important will be missing. You'll have what is known in journalism as a "hole" in your story. For a reader searching for information, finding more holes than pertinent material can be painful.

Therefore, I maintain that a journalistic approach to any form of writing is the fastest and most accessible way to tackle even a master's thesis or doctoral dissertation. I have devoted this informal but comprehensive book to you who work mainly as health caregivers and professionals, and I hope you don't find yourself "reeling" as you go through it. During the course of my research in order to devise a fresh, unorthodox "slice of writing," I wrote the book by taking into account your needs and aspirations and what anyone who wants to write should know, from common mistakes to deep-seated fears of "putting it in writing."

My mission, I believe, is to offer you—who are busy, perhaps preoccupied, stressed, and often too exhausted to dot another "i"—a guidebook that has something useful and entertaining on every page. You can open this book anywhere and, I hope, pick up a good tip on writing that nursing, social work, physical or occupational therapy or other article you've been meaning to write for eons. Or the book that's churning within you.

If nothing else, let *Toward Painless Writing* serve as your "wake-up call" to writing, a cheer for empowerment, the conquest of what you thought was impossible to achieve. The present, the gift that is here and now, is truly all we ever have. Therefore, it seems exactly the time to go for the gold.

But in going for the gold, I don't necessarily believe in "no pain, no gain." Rather, I lean toward author and New Age guru Stuart Wilde's idea that if too much of a struggle, too much pain, characterizes a situation, it may not be the correct path for you at the moment. Wilde proclaims that life doesn't have to be a struggle, and I maintain that writing doesn't have to be either. To reiterate, it's all a matter of attitude adjustment—letting go instead of retaining a dread of putting something in writing; developing an ease for self-expression as opposed to protecting self-consciousness and inhibition.

As an author of a book on writing skills, I decided to let go of convention and become an open book to my readers by offering some of my successful and my miserable experiences. I may be the "bad girl" of all the writing texts —the renegade who sticks with the fact that there are dozens of ways to do something and a better way after that and a better way after that, as Earl Nightingale said many years ago in his self-empowerment lectures. I believe if you are a health professional who realizes the value of learning from other professionals' ideas and experiences, you can make this book work for you. I also believe in the power of "baby steps," "manageable bites," or however you might characterize the condensation of an infinite topic into smaller, more understandable parts.

Certainly, if I can write about health care and related topics, so can you. Why not reach out? The world is waiting for you. It is a matter of willingness to get over the "mountain" of resistance that often knocks the pen out of your hand. The "mountain" is really just a speed bump. Simply decide to write. Be willing. The same principle applies to the clients you care for—they must first be willing to seek and accept care and participate in their own care.

Putting your knowledge and thoughts out for your colleagues and others of many disciplines is a fine thing to do; it is akin to setting up a banquet for people to experience and enjoy. The time I spend reading journal articles and books by health professionals creates in me great motivation, inspiration, and a sense of caregiver unity, which I believe is not only fundamentally good for caregivers, but excellent for our becoming a more compassionate and spiritual species on Earth. You who have already written have brought much enrichment to my life as a writer, so please continue. You who are about to write will no doubt find a new satisfaction that enhances your job and your entire profession. Please step forward.

In order to provide you the friendliest, most comprehensible assistance, I've elected to include the wisdom of other writers, short and not-so-short "takes" on the writing life, tips for the future writer, some of my personal ideas and predicaments, tough stances on matters such as clarity and accessibility, and anecdotes that illustrate and make memorable the tenets of professional writing. There. I hope I've given you a good swift kick, because I believe in you and in all of us. No more writhing. Let the literature begin!

Chapter 1
On the Importance of Writing

Writing for Your Professional Life

In her wonderful booklet, *Write Now: Maintaining a Creative Spirit While Homebound and Ill*, Susan Dion, PhD, said: "Writing (creative thinking) is a life vest. Picture it in a most vivid orange as you put it on. It will provide buoyancy as you confront the waves of a rough sea. Writing is a singular lifeline because it carries the unique thought of your personhood. It is YOU. And, preserving you is very important... Writing is life-affirming."

Take Mental Notes on Everything

Being a writer even on an occasional basis means taking mental notes on everything people say to you—for future use, of course. My children, relatives, co-workers, friends, and acquaintances have been surprised (and sometimes appalled) to read their words lifted from a casual conversation. I unabashedly pilfer bits of conversation from strangers, too, if they are within earshot and say something colorful. Health caregivers and their fields are fascinating. In sum, anyone anywhere potentially makes "good copy." Good copy is what breathes life into a book, whether it is a how-to book, a journal article, or a textbook.

Respect the Written Language

I have revered books since I was a child; few things in life receive as much of my respect and gratitude as books do. The printed word always held power—the power to enter your mind, compel you to regroup some of your old ideas, and plug in new, perhaps outrageous, ones. But too many of us become giddy at the very idea of writing. Why, articles and books drop from the Great Beyond only onto the stardusted heads of geniuses, right? Oh, please! The second President of the United States, John Adams, said, "Let us dare to read, think, speak, and write." To my mind, he meant all of us.

The Authoritative Look of Print

An experiment I did as a teenager proved memorable. I'd been wrestling with the notion that my writing would never measure up to that of the excellent published authors. So, to see if I could boost my confidence, I typed a page of William Golding's *Lord of the Flies*, which I thought astounding in style and content.

The result amused me for all time: the typewritten page did not look as authoritative and awe-inspiring as the printed page of the book. This is not to say Golding's text lost its value. Rather, the typed page, with its clumsily corrected mistakes helped me realize I always judged my work too harshly when I compared it to published literature. Instead of feeling defeated each time I pulled a typed sheet of paper from beneath the ribbon, I became aware that a hand-typed page just didn't look polished.

Today's personal computer technology affords a writer a variety of fonts, some of which look typeset, as they would in a book. If you are fortunate enough to have a computer and a high-quality printer, you're off to a better start than I had as a writer. You can see immediately the impact your copy—that is, your own prose—has on a page. Does it command you to read it? Wonderful. "Stage presence" helps a lot.

Writing Is as Easy as Bleeding

You've heard it a thousand times: elders, long-suffering spouses, blowhards, and innocents who have survived harrowing life experiences boil things down in their minds to: "I could write a book!" Why not be someone who really does just that, especially if you have been inspired by the writing of other health professionals?

The answer: most of us fear both peer and professional criticism. The philosopher Elbert Hubbard said: "To avoid criticism, do nothing, say nothing, be nothing." Some claim writing is a snap because all you need is a pencil and paper and voilà! Nothing to it. Sportswriter Red Smith said writing is easy: "All you do is sit down at the typewriter and open a vein."

Use Your Imagination Even in Academic and Nonfiction Writing

Best-selling author Michael Crichton is a MD who realized his incredible imagination took him far beyond his skill as a physician. For us less luminous caregiving folk, the message is to let our imagination have its say at least once in a while.

No Time to Write?

Many health professionals long to write about their patients and experiences. Some practitioners have new or radical ideas that could turn into provocative literature in their field, but the mere thought of spending all that time and struggling with spelling and grammar and confronting a computer word-processing program and what to say first and what not to say and how to say things so they sound really professional and doing a bibliography and writing cover letters to publishers and then on top of everything getting mixed or bad reviews as a reward for such torture, well, whew! It's just too much after a long day's journey into health care. This, dear colleagues, is a tragedy, because we need you to share the details of that journey with us.

Products of Passion

Health professionals with a passion for their work can and must add writing to their list of priorities. Passion, I say again. What a shame it would have been if Florence Nightingale had not made the time (notice made and not found) to write her ideas on how to run a hospital and care for the infirm. Her *Notes on Nursing* triggered inspiration for literature that is still viable and profound for students in health care fields. What if Marie Curie hadn't created a careful account of her work?

Think of the important movers and shakers in your field: Sister Elizabeth Kenny, the Australian nurse and physiotherapist; Dr. C. F. Samuel Hahnemann, the German physician who developed homeopathy; Galen and Hippocrates, the Ancient Greek physicians and writers; and many others. Spokespersons all, and thank heaven for their documentation and/or others' documentation of them and their work.

Reassurance Is Always Welcome

At a meeting at Robert Wood Johnson Medical Center in New Brunswick, NJ, where I was on assignment to do a nursing ethics article, about 15 nurses around the conference table identified themselves and their work one by one. As a reporter, I expected only to be a fly on the wall.

But to my surprise, I was asked to identify myself. I said I was a registered nurse working full-time as a journalist, and I remember feeling sheepish—that somehow I strayed from the flock—in the presence of all the practicing nurses. One nurse picked up on my discomfort and announced her delight that I was there. "Nursing needs spokespersons," she said to me in front of the entire group. "We need you."

Teach Unabashedly

Mexican author Carlos Fuentes explained, "Reading, writing, teaching, learning are all activities aimed at introducing civilizations to each other." This is especially applicable to health care fields. Professional health care is a tremendous, complex civilization always hungry for new literature, a new twist on a rock-solid method, and original thinking—the kind that leads to greater knowledge, cures for diseases, and better preventive measures.

Start With a Loving Desire to Write

Writer Annie Dillard offers this anecdote: A well-known writer got collared by a university student who asked, "Do you think I could be a writer?"

"Well," the writer said, "I don't know... Do you like sentences?"

The writer could see the student's amazement. Sentences? Do I like sentences? I am 20 years old and do I like sentences? If he had liked sentences, of course, he could begin, like a joyful painter I knew. I asked him how he came to be a painter. He said, "I liked the smell of the paint."

Let's get down to brass tacks. I love words. I love etymology. I love sentences. Do you like sentences and your chosen field enough to put pen to paper? If you've read this far, you probably do. Your desire to write propels you to your first sentence; all writing is, of course, is a lot of sentences strung together in an intelligent way to give information and create an enriching mental image for the reader.

Use a Computer, Typewriter, or Pen, as Long as You Use Your Ability to Write

As far as I can tell, the writer's best friends are a computer and user-friendly software. Many word-processing programs work well. Most publishers of journals, books, and other publications prefer letter-quality print-outs (as opposed to dot-matrix) and programs that are either updated to accommodate their computer software or convertible to their software, such as ASCII (a universal software program).

Be prepared to send the publisher both hard copy (your printout) and a copy of the computer disk.

Some diehards still prefer a typewriter (or claim they do, anyway), or even a pen and pad on which to write longhand because of the poetic "feel," the directness, of the pen in hand. Nonetheless, publishers won't read long-hand items, and typewriters don't yield the ever-sought-after floppy disk. Whatever mechanics one prefers, a writer uses everything available to him or her and gets the work to the publisher in a clean, acceptable format. If you are not computer literate, you can get software that comes with its own tutorial and/or a manual that explains all the functions of the computer program, such as how to double space, indent paragraphs, italicize words, save copy, print copy, etc.

Confidentiality in Health Care Writing

Sometimes the information you receive on a topic is "off the record." However, privacy and confidentiality can be maintained by altering names and situations. If a person or organization specifically tells you not to print a certain piece of information, **honor that request**.

If You Can Say It, You Can Write It

My son, a drummer, recently studied West African drumming and percussion with a respected Nigerian musician named Babatunde Olatunji. "Baba," as he is called, taught a rhythm based on three words that sound like "gun go do (pronounced "doe"), gun go do." "If you can say it," Baba said, "you can play it." The sound you make with your mouth mimics the sound you can get from the drum with your hand.

In this light, I contend that if you can confer with a colleague on a patient's history, if you can tell a joke, chances are good you can write it. You can write an article. And if you can write an article, you may well be able to stretch into a book.

Hearing What You Write

Read your written work aloud to yourself so you can **hear** it. Is it fluid and melodious? Choppy? Stiff? Change it until it sounds right to you and sounds like you. "Your material is your self," said writing expert William Zinsser.

Reading Teaches You to Write

Read, read, read. Read anything that catches your attention. I read book after book when I was a child, often saving up lunch money to buy books the strait-laced librarians wouldn't let me take out of the library. *The Nun's Story*, by Kathryn Hulme, was so well-crafted a story about a nurse/missionary nun it made me want to write. Perhaps it even encouraged me to become a nurse. (I also toyed with the idea of joining a convent, but scrapped it once reality set back in.)

So What if Your Name Isn't Hemingway?

Remember: Matthew, Mark, Luke, and John—all simple souls—did not hesitate to write (or have some scribe write) their versions of the teachings of Jesus. I daresay not one of them had any lofty ideas about professional journals, peer reviews, agents, best-sellers, or movie rights. Most points of view are worth hearing and writing. So just do it—write now.

You Don't Need to Put on Airs in Writing

Brenda Ueland wrote a wonderful book entitled *If You Want to Write*. This is one of many memorable passages: "Yes, you must feel when you write, free. You must disentangle all oughts. You must disconnect all shackles, weights, obligations, all duties. You can write as badly as you want to. You can write anything you want to, a six-act blank verse, symbolic tragedy, or a vulgar short story. Just so that you write it with honesty and gusto, and do not try to make somebody believe that you are smarter than you are. What's the use? You can never be smarter than you are. You try to be and everybody sees through it like glass, and on top of that knows you are lying and putting on airs. (Though remember this: while your writing can never be brighter, greater than you are, you can hide a shining personality and gift in a cloud of dry, timid writing.)"

Ueland also advises never to write like an advertising writer, even though she said they are among the cleverest, wittiest people. She objects to writing meant only to impress people, "convince them something is very fine about which (the writer) himself does not really care a button." I cannot imagine a health professional not caring about what he or she has chosen to write. Your caring will withstand any small violations of writing "rules"; caring will always surface.

Be Open to Your Accumulated Experience as a Caregiver

As a caregiver, and at times a care recipient, you're always risking success and failure as your writing seems to expose you to your colleagues. Hara Estroff Marano, editor of *Psychology Today*, wrote: "It's a whole-body charge when you succeed. You'd just as soon crawl under a desk when you don't." My advice here is take the chance. It won't kill you, and it may do others some good.

Chapter 2
On Getting Started

Write What You Know

You've been bombarded with this idea, of course, but I must tell you at least once in this book. This does not mean you are not allowed to select a topic you know little about and thoroughly research it. It means that after you've researched something, you know about it and can therefore write about it. However, the ideas, values, and circumstances that shape your life may be the best fodder you'll ever have.

Only you can describe an experience that moved or changed you; you were there and you know. As lawyer and author Gerry Spence put it, "You are your own authority." Give what you truly know to your readers. Now more than ever, many professional journals give space to personal stories from which other professionals can benefit. As difficult as some publishers may seem, they want manuscripts that tell true and powerful stories.

Write a First Sentence That Compels the Reader to Read On

A good start to an article (or any piece) translates into "journalese" as the "lead." The lead is so named because it leads the reader, or rather, lures the reader, into the web you are weaving. Your goal is to hook a reader into your train of thought immediately and keep him or her hooked to the end of the story unless he or she has to perform a Heimlich maneuver on someone who is choking on a chicken bone.

I am convinced that journalistic techniques such as the lead will help you the most no matter what you are writing—even an in-house memorandum. There isn't one form of writing that can't benefit from having the writer use the five Ws. The best result of employing the five Ws as a basis for all forms of professional writing is that you are forced to organize: State your case, recount and explain the aspects of your case, include who says what about the case, and come to some conclusion that is clear and satisfying.

Choose a Manageable Topic

Narrow a broad topic, such as "physical therapy," down to a more manageable topic, such as "new uses of hydrotherapy for the pediatric patient." When your mother told you as a child not to shove the whole piece of cake into your mouth at once, she was giving advice applicable to your professional career. Better to understand and savor a perfect sliver than to choke on a generous wedge.

Model Leads That Can Help Get You Started

Here are some leads from articles I've written over the years. You may find them useful as models:

- **For a feature on preventive eye care:** "Them There Eyes," those marvelous little spheres that give and receive a world of information, can last a lifetime with proper care and preventive measures. But as a rule, we don't often think of making our eyes more comfortable.
- **For a review of a plastic surgeon's book:** Dr. Robert M. Goldwyn's *Beyond Appearance: Reflections of a Plastic Surgeon* is the treatment of choice for anyone who has felt skeptical or even hostile toward a physician.
- **For a report on babies who need pacemakers:** Though a child may seem to be in "perpetual motion," he may be one of many who suffer from complete congenital heart block or other heart-rhythm irregularities, treatable by an artificial pacemaker.
- **For a report on hernia repair:** Beware the hernia: a lump in the groin, around the umbilicus (navel), or a protrusion at the site of an old surgical incision.
- **For a report on the need for organs for transplantation:** Leaving one's body—parts or all—

to science has become a well-known phrase but not a common action. What is happening to one of the most life-saving harvests of our time?

- **For a story on an enterostomal therapist:** Most people think of E.T. as Hollywood's extra-terrestrial. But Cheryl Scavron is an E.T.—enterostomal therapist—dealing with down-to-earth problems of ostomy patients.
- **For a story on chiropractic:** During the infancy of healing arts, one might have had his head "trephined"—holes bored in the skull to release evil spirits—in the event of headaches. As analgesics are ever-strengthening, it is time to re-evaluate the effectiveness of chiropractic for relief of pain and health problems.

You've got the hang of it by now. Don't be afraid to start.

Try the Free Association Technique

When I come up with an idea for an article or book, I free associate. You can use free association to help you start on a health report, journal article, thesis, or other form of writing. For example, if you're an occupational therapy student doing a paper on Post-Traumatic Stress Disorder, you might list the following words or phrases: War is hell; distress vs. eustress; following orders; trauma center; veterans administration hospitals; inappropriately abrasive speech; fear of death; guilt; grief; rehabilitation; and so on.

Free association is productive and gives you an overall handle on a subject. You'd be surprised at how effective this method is when you think you don't know a darn thing about a subject or how to begin.

The Writer's Arsenal Starts With a Dictionary

Have dictionary, will travel. You'll need at least one good dictionary, such as *Merriam Webster's Collegiate Dictionary* (the latest edition), for general English usage; a medical dictionary, such as *Taber's* or *Dorland's*; *Quick Reference Dictionary for Occupational Therapy* by Dr.

Karen Jacobs may be helpful; a thesaurus (for those
moments you're hell-bent on finding a sexier word for
something than the simple, direct one you already have);
and any other references that pertain to your field or
subject. A comprehensive encyclopedia works wonders,
too, especially for background information that can bolster
your health articles as well as your novel. Some computer
software offers medical and health-related references on
CD-ROM.

Keep It Simple

You don't need a huge vocabulary in order to write well.
Rather, you need to master the words you already know
and set them spinning your gold. There's no point in
discounting the simplest way to say something. Simplicity
is an art. Too often people believe they will sound dull,
dumb, or unprofessional if they do not use big words and
complex sentences.

What had long been considered "academic style," that
is, literature written for intellectuals in a particular field,
has all but taken a flying leap into oblivion. This is not to
say that writing should not be intellectual or geared to
intellectual thinking, nor is it to say that a writer should
never use a polysyllabic or technical word. Instead, the
emphasis falls on clarity and accessibility of the work.

Some of my favorite writers—M. Scott Peck, Carolyn
Myss, Robert Coles, Robert Hughes, Deepak Chopra,
Wayne Dyer, Anne Lamott, Colleen McCullough, Kathryn
Hulme, and others—construct their sentences with
amazing grace. They avoid fillers and puffery and favor
directness. In that directness lies the force of their ideas.
William Zinsser advocates using words you normally use in
everyday speech. If you're not one to say "indeed," leave it
out of your writing.

Ask Research Experts for Help

Reference librarians are enormously helpful. They can
get you started on researching a topic, and they can bail you
out of trouble when you hit a snag. I've called many a

librarian to ask who wrote the "Happy Birthday to You" song, how to spell portobello, as in portobello mushrooms, and other weird questions. They tend to go out of their way for you either on the telephone or in person at the library. Don't forget to acknowledge them.

The Joy of the Active Voice

Start with an active voice. Rise B. Axelrod and Charles R. Cooper, authors of *The St. Martin's Guide to Writing,* contend that "(s)ome writers use passives to give a false impression of scientific objectivity or to hide the actor's identity and thereby avoid responsibility for the action. Because of the verbal smoke screen that passives construct, they are popular within impersonal institutions and large bureaucracies and with those who seek to defend the indefensible: Action to clean up toxic waste sites was not taken....Last year it was recommended by the student government that a board of review be created to that students would be given a greater voice in campus governance."

When you use the passive voice—"was not taken," "it was recommended," etc.—you clutter and weaken your sentences. Better to write "No one cleaned up the toxic waste sites," and "Last year the student government recommended that the school create a board of review to give students a greater voice in campus governance."

Look at What Has Already Been Published on Your Topic

I learned to write by reading. I did not major in journalism or English, but I learned the principles of journalism by reading the daily newspaper and imitating the structure of its articles. Eventually, I developed my own style using journalism's well-established techniques.

Look for and study models. If you want to write a book about physical therapy techniques, for example, gather all the books you can find on that subject to see what has already been done and how. In the library, check the listing of books and articles in print on the subject. Then decide on your approach.

Writing Is Compatible With Any Occupation or Profession

Writing is compatible with any line of work. One successful novelist works full-time as a longshoreman. He says a more intellectually demanding day job would interfere with his creativity. You can be a butcher, baker, or candlestick-maker and write. So why think your job as a social worker, nurse, or therapist precludes writing?

Organize Your Ideas

Most people think you must start with a formal outline, Roman numerals and all. This may work for you just wonderfully, but it never really worked for me. I think it is easier to make that kind of outline of a piece after it is finished. However, you do need to organize your thoughts. Getting them on paper helps you assess, evaluate, order, and re-order them.

You can do this by writing the first sentence, saying exactly what you want to say, and taking it from there. Move logically from one point to another, increasing the power of your lead or "thesis statement." Or you can have a private brainstorming session and jot down all the points you wish to make in an article or book. Organize them and see to it their order makes sense. Use the "Sesame Street" system. Segments of this popular children's show address the concept of logical order, i.e., what happens next? Once your ideas and premises are well-placed, you can expand and explain each one.

Center Yourself

Before you start writing, turn off the radio, television, telephone, and anything else that can mar your thoughts. Learn to connect your inner voice with the words you intend to share with the outside world. Many writers meditate, or get quiet, in some way. If you try to do a term paper while watching Oprah, both activities will suffer.

Give the term paper your full attention. Doing one thing at a time is not the typical way of our mad-rush culture, but I recommend it highly, especially for writing.

In addition, don't run off and elope with your first sentence. It may not be the best approach. Sometimes you can fall in love with how you are saying something, but you may be the only one who understands it. I remember doing an elaborate feature on an artist for an arts magazine and having the editor rake it over the coals. Rewriting it, I eliminated all the hocus-pocus I thought sounded "artistic." I replaced passive verbs with active ones and realized the strength and dignity of "he said" as opposed to "he gestured wildly." It wasn't the best story I ever wrote, but the revised version offered the reader much cleaner access to the artist and his work.

The same concept can apply to an anecdotal health feature such as the ones found in nursing and other journals, and it can apply to more technical pieces that often favor needless jargon or complication.

In any case, refuse to be intimidated by anyone who tells you you're no Shakespeare. Scholars are still arguing about whether Shakespeare was Shakespeare. If you have something valuable to share with readers, then write it as simply and directly as possible. An Irish proverb applies to would-be but reluctant writers: "The bird that can sing and won't sing should be made to sing."

What to Do When You Can't Think of What to Write

Can't seem to come up with an idea? There are books in the library, such as *10,000 Ideas for Term Papers, Projects, Reports, and Speeches*, so no excuses. It's like health care: When you need relief from pain, you seek it. You may find that the simplest idea works out the best.

The Good, the Bad, and the Ugly in Writing on Health Care

In his book *Writing Creative Nonfiction*, Theodore A. Rees Cheney says in researching a topic, you should be willing to dig into "that which smells bad (as well as that which smells wonderful) and listen to that which repels (as well as that with which you agree). All this sensory acquisition will provide the concrete and sensory details you'll need to create for your reader the objective reality of the situation. You'll need, too, to dig deep into the emotional side of those interviewed, finding out their innermost thoughts and feelings, if you're to give your readers that subjective reality, which, when combined artfully with the objective reality, will paint for them as honest and accurate a picture of the world as it's possible for you, a fallible human, to paint." Truth is eternal. Write the truth.

Chapter 3
On Words

Good, Strong Words

I've always cherished the character of Jo March in *Little Women*. Her sisters would criticize her for her expletives, the worst of which was "Blast!" But as an aspiring writer, she countered, "I like good strong words that mean something!" Bear that in mind when you write about a patient's endurance of a disease process, or about the therapist who feels burned out on the job, or about a new theory on pain management. Again, the simplest word is usually the strongest.

Help the Reader "Experience" What You're Writing About

Dr. Wayne W. Dyer's book *You'll See It When You Believe It* begins with an intriguing concept of words: "You cannot drink the word 'water.' The formula H_2O cannot float a ship. The word 'rain' cannot get you wet. You must experience water or rain to truly know what the words mean. Words themselves keep you several steps removed from the experience. And so it is with everything that I write about in this book. These are words that are meant to lead to the direct experience. If the words I write ring true, it is very likely that you will take the ideas presented here and create your experience of them."

In his book *The Writer's Art* James J. Kilpatrick wrote: "We tend to conclude that people who use words with which we happen not to be familiar are using unfamiliar words. If John knows 8,000 words and Susan knows 8,000 words, inevitably John will know 250 words that Susan does not, and Susan will know 250 words that John does not, and John will think Susan exhibitionistic, and Susan will think John affected... but I think that writers have an obligation to keep the frontiers of language open... "

Words That Are Often Misused

1. **Between and Among.** Know the difference between the words "between" and "among." Between refers to placement in the middle of two things, e.g., "between a rock and a hard place," "between New York and Los Angeles." You cannot be between three or more things, however. You can be in the midst of things, so use "among," e.g., "She walked among us," and "He has written many books, *The Return of Merlin* among them." This is a controversial issue and involves several subtleties in usage.
    Follow the dictionary's rules or make a judgment about how a sentence works best. I would say as long as there is a separation going on, use between, e.g., "between you and me." *Webster's (10th ed.)* advocates "between you and me and the lamppost." I advise you not to lose sleep over this, in any case.
2. **That.** Eliminate superfluous "thats." "The book that I am writing" tightens up nicely as "The book I am writing." Same meaning, leaner sentence. Remember to "write tight."
3. **Hopefully.** Let's all stop saying and writing, "Hopefully, I'll get the job done." This use of "hopefully" is ungrammatical. What you mean is, "I hope I'll get the job done" or "It is hoped the job will get done." Hopefully does not mean "I hope." It means "in a hopeful manner," according to *The Associated Press Stylebook and Libel Manual*, and it is not interchangeable with "let us hope," "we hope," or "it is hoped."
4. **Sexist Words.** Avoid sexist usage, such as "comedienne" and "actress." Nowadays women prefer to be known as comedians and actors. Dietitian, not dietician. Avoid stewardess (now all are called flight attendants), waitress ("server" is a better, non-sexist term), etc. Also, non-sexist language is so preferred that a grammatical error is now well-

accepted in spoken and written English: "Everyone has their opinion." Everyone is a singular subject, so by rights it takes a singular possessive pronoun, his or her. You should say, "Everyone has his or her opinion," but using his and her all the time seems cumbersome. "Their" is a plural possessive pronoun, but it has gained great favor in this context. Guardians of the English language, swallow hard! As the Irish say, "You cannot force the sea."

5. **Words You Can't Spell.** Remember Anne Bancroft's portrayal of Annie Sullivan in "The Miracle Worker" when Annie wanted to know how to spell "discipline?" She said how ridiculous it was that you had to know how to spell it before you could look it up to find out how to spell it!

6. **Jargon and Esoteric Terms.** One of my editors came to my desk with a hot head. She was wild because I used the word "scumble" in my art column. "We can't use that word. You made it up!" she said. "I did not," I said. "It's an art term meaning to soften the lines of a drawing." She then said it was not in the dictionary and therefore could not stand in the story. But, to her dismay, it was in the dictionary we all used. "Well, don't send readers to the dictionary!" she grumbled and stalked off. I should have told her I frequently read the dictionary just for fun. So do lots of other people.

7. **Jive and Jibe.** To jibe means to fit in with or go along with something; don't use the word "jive" when you mean jibe. For example, "The therapist's frown did not jibe with her encouraging words." The noun jive means slang, foolish or teasing talk, or swing music and dancing.

8. **Try.** Yoda, a character in the film "The Empire Strikes Back," says, "No such thing as try. Only do or not do." This is a terrific way to remember the difficulties inherent in using the word "try" when you can probably substitute a better verb. "The physician tried to do all he could for the patient" reads more concisely as "The physician did all he could for the

patient." Try often seems superfluous. Also, many people say, "Try and read this sentence." "Try and" is overkill; better to write, "Try to read this sentence."

9.   **When to Use Numerals Instead of Words.** Write out numbers zero through nine; use numerals for 10 and beyond. You may overload a sentence by writing "eleven hundred items on hand" as opposed to the visually friendlier "1100 items on hand." The same applies to money. Write "$4 million" instead of "four million dollars."

10.   **When to Capitalize or Use Lowercase.** Capitalize all trade names, such as Valium, and lowercase generic names, such as diazepam. Capitalize proper nouns (names), the word I, and the first word of every sentence.

11.   **Brand Names.** Unless you don't mind advertising a product or using a colloquial term, avoid brand names in your articles. Use bandages instead of "Band-Aids," and doughnuts instead of "Dunkin' Donuts." Remember that everyday use of a brand name instead of its generic name and common mispronunciations may lead to incorrect spelling.

12.   **A While, A Lot, All Right.** She will arrive in a while. Not in "awhile." The client learned a lot from the therapist. Not "alot." The nurse said things would be all right. Not "alright."

13.   **Different From.** When you want to point out differences, write different from, not different than, which is extremely popular but ungrammatical. One thing is different from another. "His story is different from her story."

14.   **When to Use Italics and Quotation Marks.** Italicize foreign words, such as *joie de vivre*, and genus and species, such as *Cannabis sativa* (hemp); italicize book titles and words used for emphasis; put quotation marks around titles of articles, movies, plays, and what people actually say—word for word. Some writers believe people's grammatical errors and linguistic idiosyncrasies should be written as they are spoken, such as "He went to da terlet." (Or is it

spelled "turlet"?) Certainly novelists take great pains to recreate a dialect or accent because it adds vibrance to their characters. When caregivers write about patients or others they encounter in their daily work, why "clean up" a person's colorful speech in false deference to written language? Isn't it more engaging to have a vivid image of a person, such as, "So you believe it's God's will, is it?" as opposed to "You believe it is God's will?" The whitewashed version lacks personality and takes character away from the speaker. However, if a person uses objectionable words, you'll have to decide, according to the publication and audience for which you are writing, whether to indicate each expletive by a letter and dashes, use the words as they were spoken, or eliminate them altogether.

15. **Quirky Spellings.** Minuscule, not miniscule; gray, not grey. Paying attention to details counts more than you think.

16. **Proper Names.** Make sure you always spell proper names correctly. One of the first rules of journalism is to get the person's name right. Think how you feel whenever someone misspells your name. Also remember: Smithsonian Institution, not Institute, Johns Hopkins University, not John Hopkins, etc. Spelling is like pouring medications: Check, double check, and triple check before administering drugs to the patient, and after you administer the drug, check it again before you put it away.

17. **Plural Forms.** Cupfuls is the correct plural, as is mothers-in-law. One editor inserted "theirself," instead of "themselves," into one of my stories. I was horrified to see this in print, and I thought I should kill myself on the spot. Then I realized that anyone who knew me and my work would know some dopey editor did it. But the truth is, many people think the person with the by-line is the one responsible for whatever appears in print. Fact: Not all editors are grammarians, good spellers, or even writers, for that matter.

18. **Livid.** Livid is often used to mean "red with rage," but according to *Webster's Collegiate Dictionary*, the first two meanings are "black-and-blue," as in bruising, and "ashen" or ghostly pale. The fourth meaning is "very angry."

19. **Homonyms—Same Sound, Different Meaning.** Watch out for homonyms, words that sound the same but are spelled differently and have different meanings. For example, don't use "horde" (a swarm, throng, or crowd) if you mean "hoard" (to collect zealously and possibly to excess). "Going to the market to buy too many apples" illustrates other homonyms that are often misspelled. Common errors include there and their; weather and whether; heard and herd; cite, sight, and site; here and hear; presents and presence; past and passed; whose and who's; its and it's; knew and new; lead and led; etc.

20. **Amount and Number.** In an article in a nursing publication, the lead included the sentence, "No one knows the amount of things I do each day." Don't confuse amount and number. For example, "I have a great number of things to do today," and "There is a large amount of work to do." Amount tells you how much; number tells you how many.

21. **Over and More Than.** How acceptable the phrase "over a billion sold" has become! Too bad, because this use of "over" is ungrammatical. Instead, use more than, e.g., "More than 6,000 social workers attended the conference." When you wish to communicate a person's advanced age, use older than instead of over, e.g., "The patient was older than 65." Or, "A patient must be 65 or older to be eligible."

22. **Under and Less Than.** The same applies to "under." Write, "There were fewer than 200 applicants," not "under 200 applicants." Don't substitute under for less than or younger than. *Incorrect:* "He is under 18." *Correct:* "He is younger than 18."

23. **Continue, Off, and Where It Is.** Avoid redundancies such as "continue on" and "off of." *Incorrect:* "She continued on speaking." *Correct:*

"She continued to speak." *Incorrect:* "He pulled the sheet off of the bed." *Correct:* "He pulled the sheet off the bed." *Incorrect:* "She told me where she was at." *Correct:* "She told me where she was."

24. **That and Which.** Understand the difference between that and which. Use which when you want to add information to a sentence. Use that when the addition cannot be eliminated without changing the point of the sentence. For example, "The maternal-child clinic program, which was designed by a nurse, began today." Although interesting, the phrase "which was designed by a nurse" is not crucial to the meaning of the sentence. But, "The maternal-child clinic that began today created a stir in the community." See the different angle here?

25. **One Compound Word or Two Separate Words?** Know which words should be separate and which are compound words. For example, there is no such thing as a gall bladder, making bladder the noun and gall an adjective. The correct word, a noun, is gallbladder. Eyestrain, headache, backache, toothache, earache, nosebleed, etc., are compound words. If a word you suspect may be compound is not in the dictionary, most likely it is not compound, but two separate words. The dictionary lists all compound words, some separate words that are frequently used together, such as foul play, and hyphenated words, such as cross-eye (strabismus).

26. **Counterfeit, or "Weasel" Words.** Counterfeit words, according to Edmond H. Weiss, author of *The Writing System for Engineers and Scientists*, should be avoided: "preventative" instead of preventive; "administrate" instead of administer; "orientate" instead of orient, "irregardless" instead of regardless, "firstly" instead of first, "deselect" instead of reject, etc.

27. **Due to and Because Of.** Weiss also demonstrates the difference between "due to" and "because of": "There is a strange phobia in America about beginning a

sentence with because...Again, there is simply no such rule!

No: Due to the strike, our installation was delayed.

Yes: Because of the strike our installation was delayed.

No: Due to a number of user mistakes, we are rewriting our manual.

Yes: Because of the number of user mistakes, we are rewriting our manual.

Yes: The replacement of our manual is due to the number of user errors."

Use due to, Weiss advises, only as a synonym for attributable to and only after the verb to be (is, are, was, were, be) or after another "linking verb" (seems, appears.)

28. **More.** "More's the pity": Watch out for saying "more better" instead of better, "more healthy" instead of healthier, "more free" instead of freer.

29. **"Manufractured" Words.** It may not sound fair, but I hate the word "humongous." It's in the same category as "discombobulated" and "thingamajig." Use this type of word for color and in direct quotes, but choose wisely.

30. **Polite Words.** I agree with Edmond Weiss on the phrases of politeness that have become standard in our writing, especially in professional memos and letters. They are meant to sound warm and sincere, but they come across as false and cold and, well, standard. For example: Enclosed please find...Do not hesitate to call...We regret any inconvenience...You are cordially invited...It's been a pleasure...I certainly hope...It was a pleasant experience...We are experiencing difficulties...

31. **Enormity.** One of my pet peeves has been overruled by *Webster's (10th ed.)*, and I'm not a good sport about it. I maintain that enormity does not refer to the size of something; enormity means evil or wickedness—the enormity of his crime, for example. Many use enormity to mean enormous, vast, or huge.

Webster's says they may do so in certain contexts. Look it up before you use it.

32. **Words That Say Precisely What You Mean.** A colleague of mine told me of a man who was asked at a meeting to "approach the rectum" instead of the "lectern." Get the word right. Look it up. Do not assume you know it. According to "The Odd Couple" character Felix Unger, portrayed by Tony Randall on TV, to "ASSUME makes an ASS of U and ME."

In *The Writer's Art*, James Kilpatrick quotes the beloved American author: " 'That should always be our goal,' as Mark Twain has reminded us, 'to use the right word, and not its second cousin.' When we read that a 'house has been robbed,' we are meeting a second cousin, for houses are burglarized; people are robbed." Kilpatrick continues: "When we read that a 'partially nude' body has been found, we experience an imperceptible hesitation—for nude is just that; it is synonymous with naked, and we would not write of a 'partially naked' body. The right word in this instance would be partially clad."

33. **Lay and Lie.** He was lying down on the bed. He asked if he could lie down on the couch. Neither of these sentences should use "lay." However: Lay the pieces down on the table. He was laid to rest. Lay usually refers to placement; lie in this instance means to assume a reclining position. Remember the proverb: "You made your bed, now lie in it."

34. **Past Forms of Drown and Spay.** Past tenses of the verbs "to drown" and "to spay" are drowned, not "drownded," and spayed, not "spaded." I once heard a woman call her evening gown a "gownd," as though it were a past participle. It reminded me of the child who called the hair over her eye sockets "eyebrowns." Please be careful about quirky words that many people mispronounce and thereafter write incorrectly.

35. **Faze and Phase.** It did not faze me one bit. She is just going through an adolescent phase. Faze means affect; phase refers to a segment or time period.

36. **Very, Very Extraordinary.** From a hit song of the 1970s: "Our house is a very, very, very fine house." Very works in the song for rhythm and texture, but you can usually edit it out of your writing. For example, "very beautiful" seems somehow less believable than "beautiful." Most of the time, "beautiful" and other adjectives do nicely on their own. Also remember that what seems "very beautiful" to you may be semi-beautiful to someone else. Do not use very with unique, true, universal, imperative, unanimous, essential, dead, virgin, total, fatal, complete, indispensable, and other words that need no modifier. Something cannot be very unique; it is either unique or not. The same applies to quite, rather, and a little bit, e.g., quite pregnant, rather pregnant, a little bit pregnant.

37. **Nerve-racking, etc.** As a self-appointed member of the "spelling police," I always found it nerve-racking to see this adjective written "nerve-wracking." Then I saw a furniture store advertising "cushens," a marina's sign that offered fishing and "crabing," and a luncheonette selling "omlets." Nowadays, spelling errors abound and top each other. I believe, along with many professional writers, that correct spelling shows you care about your work and the importance of consistent word usage. If everyone started spelling words phonetically or however they liked to spell them, written English would fall apart, and its universality of meaning would erode.

38. **Typographical Errors.** Two of my favorite typographical errors of all time appeared in *The New York Times* classified section: "PUBIC RELATIONS" and "POOFREADER WANTED."

39. **Who and Whom.** Proper use of who and whom gives many of us a royal pain. Just remember that WHO is subjective and WHOM is objective. *Incorrect:* Who do you want to speak to? *Correct:* To whom (objective) do you want to speak? *Incorrect:* Whomever took my pen, please return it. *Correct:* Whoever (subjective) took my pen...

The rules pertaining to who and whom have gone astray of late, even on talk shows and news reports. Who prevails because Americans often fear using whom; they think it sounds peculiar.

40. **Whence, Herein, Herewith, Wherefore.** Whence means "from what place, source, or cause. Therefore, you do not need to say "from whence." It's redundant. Herein and herewith are obsolete businessese.
    Worthwhile trivia: In "Romeo and Juliet," Juliet says, "Wherefore art thou Romeo?" Wherefore means why, not where. She is asking not "Where are you, Romeo?" She asks why he is a Montague. Now, don't you feel better to have that straight? I do. There's nothing like taking moronic pleasure in having pontificated on a word nobody uses anymore.

41. **Amongst, Whilst, Oncet, and Obsolete Endings.** Amongst is an obsolete term for "among." Use among, while, once.

42. **Dangling Modifiers.** *The Associated Press Stylebook and Libel Manual* advises the writer to avoid dangling modifiers, phrases that do not refer clearly and logically to some word in the sentence:
    Dangling: Taking our seats, the game started. (Taking does not refer to the subject, game, nor to any other word in the sentence.)
    Correct: Taking our seats, we watched the opening of the game. (Taking refers to we, the subject of the sentence.)

43. **Impact, Feedback, Data, Interface, -Wise, -Ize.** Don't use the noun impact as a verb, such as "A war would impact our economy." Instead, say "A war would have an impact on our economy." Feedback is computer jargon. Data is the Latin plural of datum, so write "The data are in the file." Interface is business jargon and does not work well as a substitute for cooperate or meet or work with. A movie critic I know uses words like "movie-wise" and "budget-wise." Ugh! It reminds me of "Contrarywise" in *Alice's Adventures in Wonderland* and a character played by Jack Lemmon who says, "That's the way it

crumbles, cookie-wise." Get wise. And -ize is business jargon, too. Forget prioritize, maximize, etc. Use "to set priorities" and "make the most of" instead.

44.   **Four-Letter Words.** "Here is one reason to refrain from using four-letter words in the company of all ages, sexes, and sensibilities...it is a meretricious way of putting force in prose. (A meretrix was a Roman prostitute.) If a writer cannot shock with an original figure of speech, that writer pretends to be gutsy with the use of gutterspeak, relying on obscenity and profanity to reflect reality in dialogue. Screenwriters pepper their dialogue with street talk and project it into the theater and living room, debasing living-room talk when it is treated as acceptable by the young. As a comedian said, he was raised to think mother was half a word."—William Safire, "On Language," *The New York Times Magazine.*

Chapter 4
On Form

What Is Nonfiction?

Nonfiction refers to written material based on truth, fact, or beliefs or concepts that can be construed as fact. In other words, nonfiction means that the author is not inventing or imagining, deceiving, or falsifying any information. Forms of nonfiction include the feature story, news report, investigative report, service articles, editorial opinion, periodical article, research paper, abstract, book (often in the form of a textbook, how-to, biography, autobiography, reference, exposé, or manual), memorandum, essay (including the essay examination), thesis, dissertation, travel writing, profiles and portraits of famous people, oddities, and other people, places, and situations that have not been exposed to a wide public audience, in-house publication (newsletter, annual report, etc.), grant and other persuasive writing, business letter, speech, and in-service and workshop materials.

Blending Hard News With Feature-Writing Techniques

Terri Brooks, author of *Words' Worth: A Handbook of Writing and Selling Nonfiction,* writes: "Until recently, feature stories have had a reputation for being the soft underbelly of the news, as if they could not compete with the hard-muscled facts of newspaper journalism. But now hard-core journalists treat feature writing with more respect, and have even begun to absorb its techniques into the basic telling of the news. The truth is that features often work harder than news stories, for they add depth and perspective to events that too often seem arbitrary and serendipitous. They anchor the flight of events. And, since every feature has a 'voice,' the feature can go where hard news dare not tread, to reveal ethical and moral implications behind a breaking story. Today the best front-page stories incorporate more components of the feature: description, anecdotes, an engaging lead, lively verbs, and language made compelling not only because of the information conveyed but also because of the words used to convey it."

Health professionals may provide articles that are considered "breaking news"—the latest development or event, articles or books offering professional information, feature articles, as well as fiction based on one's experience in a certain field.

Fiction Offers Truth, Semi-Truth, and Wonderful Lies

Forms of fiction can, but need not, be based on true stories in which the truth is enhanced, exaggerated, or used as a "skeleton" upon which is fashioned a "fleshier" piece of literature. Most fiction writers use subjects they know about as a starting point for an otherwise imaginary tale.

For instance, Margaret Mitchell's one and only book, *Gone with the Wind*, centers on the Civil War and the struggles of a southern belle and her dashing man, characters based on her own marriage. Fiction forms include the short story, novel, novella, and play. Some say poetry is neither fact nor fiction, but I concur with Wallace Stevens, who wrote that "poetry is the supreme fiction." Usually the writer of fiction (and poetry, for that matter) has total charge of what transpires—he or she is, essentially, telling a fascinating "lie" or an embellished truth that may well teach us something worthwhile.

Health Literature Needs Fiction and Nonfiction

Most health writing is nonfiction—that is, written to impart information in an accessible, compelling way. (Unfortunately, not all nonfiction is compelling; think of some of the arid textbooks you had to crawl through on

your belly like a stranded French Foreign Legionnaire.)
Fictional works dealing with health topics are also valuable
and may have great impact on actual health care practice.
The recent films "Lorenzo's Oil" and "The Doctor" come to
mind, both dramatizations based on true stories. As Charles
Dickens put it in *Hard Times*: "Facts alone are wanted in
life."   And we cannot forget the 19th-century proverb,
"Truth is stranger than fiction."

Offer Your Facts Up Front

"If your research is strong, then everyone should know
it. So state what you did up front—the first paragraph, even
the first sentence—and leave the dilly-dallying for people
who don't have anything to report," says Erich Kunhardt,
quoted in *The Craft of Scientific Writing* by Michael Alley.

The Key to Strong Scientific Writing

I think Michael Alley does all health professionals who
want to improve their writing a great favor by giving us the
precise key to strong scientific writing. Alley says:

"You must inform your audience as efficiently as
possible. You must stay honest...In scientific writing,
'efficiency' does not mean the paper with the shortest
length; rather, the paper that takes the readers the shortest
time to understand. (And) being honest means including all
data points, even those that don't fit the curve. It means not
hiding flaws in your research beneath a snow bank of
complex writing. To be honest, you must give fair
treatment to opposing theories and experiments.

"Science is not religion. You must base all your
arguments on logic, not emotion....Literary writing, on the
other hand, has no single defined purpose. There can be
any number of reasons behind the writing of a poem or a
story: anger, love, depression, even boredom."

Structure Within Structure

In his book, *Writing With a Purpose*, Joseph F. Trimmer
quotes nonfiction writer John McPhee, who said that
"everything in writing is a structure within a structure

within a structure down to a simple sentence, which, of course, is also a structure."

First, Write a Coherent, Enticing Paragraph

Words hang together to make sentences, and sentences, like a series of "undergutchies" on a clothesline, make paragraphs. (I got the word "undergutchies" from an editor I worked with years ago. He prided himself on being a guardian of the English language, which indeed he was, except for liking "undergutchies" as a euphemism for underwear.) The trick is to make the reader's eye go freely from one pair of lacy drawers to another in order to understand what information you are offering.

According to Joseph F. Trimmer, "the main orders of movement within paragraphs are:

1.   General to particular. Opening general statement or topic sentence followed by illustration or details of explanation or proof. The paragraph may conclude with a restatement of the topic sentence.

2.   Particular to general. From a series of detailed statements to a conclusion drawn from them. If there is a topic sentence, it occurs at or near the end of the paragraph.

3.   Whole to parts. Paragraph begins with an introductory statement about the number of parts and then explains each part: often a first, second, third order.

4.   Question to answer, or effect to cause. Paragraph begins with question or effect, then answers the question or shows the cause."

Writing Feature Articles

"A feature story is 'soft' news, compared with the 'hard' news item that reports what has just happened, what is new, significant, and startling. The feature article is less timely than the news item but also more timeless. It rewards human curiosity...Human interest stories are feature stories focusing on people. Feature stories may also focus on problems or issues," according to Riley Hughes in *How to Write Creatively.*

Nonfiction Can Be Entertaining

Health care professionals, please take note: "Conventional nonfiction writers have usually presumed that nonfiction's purpose was not to entertain but to inform, to teach, to lecture. The latest research into how we learn, however, has found that we learn best when we are at the same time entertained, when there is a joy and pleasure in the learning," wrote Theodore A. Rees Cheney in *Writing Creative Nonfiction.*

Thirteen Ways to Begin a Story

I gave several seminars on feature writing at college symposiums. My hand-out emphasized 13 (lucky) ways to start constructing your health care feature or nonfiction piece:

1.   **Pick out a striking aspect of your subject and introduce it the way you see fit.** This is often called creating an "angle." Other information centers on the initial idea. You may have a title in mind that can spark your story. Let the article go from there. (You can also write a title last, which is what happens in the newsroom of daily papers and publishers of professional journals and other materials. Editors read, edit, and headline the stories according to the particular style of their publication and/or what their readers require.)

2.   **Begin with an interesting quote, one that tells intriguing things about your subject.** Pithy quotes are invaluable. For example, a story on the contributions of occupational therapists to the health care team might start with something Eleanor Roosevelt said:
"When you cease to make a contribution, you begin to die." (Mrs. Roosevelt would appreciate credit for the quote, of course.)

One might continue with, "When a patient's injury or illness hinders him from making his contribution, the occupational therapist can teach him ways to foil his impediment and get on with an active life."

3. **Begin with a comparison of the subject with a related idea.** For example, one medical center ran an elaborate ad campaign that told how some workers are so compassionate for their fellows that they fan them as they work in the heat. These workers and fellows, in fact, are bees, and, the ad continues, why should compassion among workers be any different at a hospital?

4. **Begin with a gathering of information that requires further explanation.** For example, "Francis Bacon, the Duke of Wellington, Henry David Thoreau, Montaigne, and Franklin D. Roosevelt have something in common besides their fame. They all expressed, in similar fashion, that 'nothing is terrible except fear itself.'" This might lead nicely into an article on anything from health care professionals' risk-taking to diagnosable phobias.

5. **Ask a question that leads into your subject.** For instance, "Is there anyone who really eats according to the recommendations of the new food pyramid?"

6. **Start with an anecdote.** Read any mainstream magazine or professional journal for a model for this structure. It's usually a case history of such universality or compelling drama that you can't ignore it.

7. **Start with a complaint or a confession**. For example, "I never realized how people's lives could be changed when a loved one becomes catastrophically ill and homebound."

8. **Set up a framework—some sort of outline or "big picture"—for your article**. Direct your information to a goal, which sometimes means writing the end first if that's the only way to recognize your goal.

9. **Pay attention to detail; leave no gaps in your information.** Make sure your reader does not finish

reading what you write with more questions than you answered. We all want to know whodunit.

10. **Keep sentences and paragraphs short, which is friendly to the eye.** Dense-looking copy with few or no indented paragraphs may be too intimidating to bother getting the magnifying glass. Shorter is usually sweeter, however, you don't want a choppy quality to your writing. Intersperse longer sentences among the short ones for a nice rhythm, which is friendly to the ear.

11. **Make good transitions.** Transition in writing is the same idea as transitions in life—pre-birth existence to birth to childhood to adulthood to death to post-death existence, and so on. Each transition holds its own characteristics and significance. Have good and logical reason for moving from one point to another. The last sentence in a paragraph should somehow link easily with the first sentence of the next paragraph.

12. **Think of your readers, your audience.** What is most important to them? How can an audience relate best to your writing, and how can your writing relate best to the audience? Start with a statement on an important, perhaps prickly, issue that provokes intense interest in your readers.

13. **Never misquote, misspell names, make grammatical errors, forget to proofread, or begin with "It was a dark and stormy night."** A good beginning to an article is like the first thing someone says that leads to an engaging conversation—just start to talk. You can always go back and polish it up if need be. Start with the best idea you have. I advise against saving your best line for the end, because there are editors who "scissor-edit," which means they lop off your last paragraph, or perhaps the last three paragraphs, to make a story fit the available space in the paper or magazine. I will talk more about editing later in this book, and I suggest you brace yourself with a vodka martini, extremely dry, straight up, with three olives.

Be an Unashamed Pest if Necessary to Get the Facts Straight

I always tell an interviewee I'd rather be a horrible pest to him or her than write something dumb or wrong. So far, no one has objected to being telephoned, even several times and twice during dinner, in the interest of accuracy.

What Is an Essay?

The essay closely resembles the "How I Spent My Summer Vacation" compositions we did in grade school: a fairly short, interpretive, personal piece adhering to one idea throughout. When autobiographical, the essay provides an oral history that is also a shared intimacy, according to Dr. Fran Weber Shaw in her book, *50 Ways to Help You Write*. Essays appear in everything from *Time* magazine to the *American Journal of Nursing*.

Professional journals are more interested in acquiring analytical and revealing essays than ever before, because essays are short but power-packed, especially when written by an astute observer or an expert in a field.

Shaw says: "Showing what happened is not reserved for fiction alone. A pertinent incident or conversation will liven up and make a strong point in any essay. You can follow the chronological order of events as they happened, or begin just before a moment of realization. Try flashing back or forward in time. Dialogue will make your writing come alive."

The essay, written to clarify or vivisect a subject for the reader's viewing pleasure, also stands as a vehicle for our understanding. As C. Day-Lewis said: "We do not write in order to be understood; we write in order to understand."

The Three Kinds of Essays

In a marvelous book for young people, *Putting It In Writing*, by Steve Otfinoski, I found the most reader-friendly explanation of the essay. The three kinds are explanatory, which is a straightforward account of something or how to do something, such as "Making Steam from Trash," or "Providing Occupational Therapy for the

Adolescent Girl"; persuasive, in which "the writer tries to persuade the reader to accept an idea or agree with an opinion" by using an engaging style and strong information that backs up the opinion; and humorous, which "takes a light-hearted look at its subject. This doesn't mean it is filled with jokes. It means that its main purpose is to entertain."

This exercise will help you decide which type of essay you need to write:

1.   Explanatory—describe the major points and details of giving your dog a flea-and-tick shampoo
2.   Persuasive—give your readers the facts about having a pet spayed or neutered and convince them that, in most cases, this is a good idea
3.   Humorous—narrate the tale of having your cat dipped, or tell a story about what happens when you give a toddler a plate of spaghetti

Talk to yourself, then write down what you say. Writing is saying—only you do it on paper.

The Four Parts of an Essay

I believe some of the clearest and most helpful information comes from books written for children. (I remember doing a critical essay on a Goya exhibition at the Metropolitan Museum of Art. I consulted the *Encyclopaedia Britannica*, which offered detailed information on the artist and his work. But it was through a children's book on the artist that I learned of Goya's physical affliction.)

Steve Otfinoski, in *Putting It In Writing*, lists the four parts of an essay as:

1.   The title, which sets the tone for the whole piece
2.   The introduction, the first paragraph that gets the reader's attention and states the writer's purpose
3.   The body, which explains or supports the main idea and is the longest part of the essay
4.   The conclusion, in which the main idea is reiterated and brought to a satisfying end

Thanks, Steve. My inner child needed that.

Your Best Essay May Be at Hand in Your Diary

Many famous writers describe their diaries or journals as a therapeutic tool, a thrusting out of their ideas and style and struggles like 100 decorated chests in a military inspection line. Keeping a diary helps you write without inhibition because it is for your eyes only. The entries give information on many levels—physical, logical, emotional, and irrational—from day to day. Often you can separate the wheat from the chaff and produce an insightful essay from your secret writings. And just think how grand it will be when your entire, unexpurgated diary is published after you're dead.

A Letter Can Serve as an Essay

A letter that provides an overview of what is happening and the emotions that accompany the situation may be an essay in the making. Never mind the "Dear, I thought I'd drop a line" stuff, but pay attention to letters that force you to think, such as the *New York Sun's* beloved "Yes, Virginia" editorial reply in 1897 by editor Francis P. Church to little Virginia O'Hanlon, who asked if there really is a Santa Claus.

I suggest you read the collected letters of excellent writers, such as the letters of Groucho Marx, or Goethe's *The Sufferings of Young Werther*, a romantic novel constructed entirely of letters, or the poignant missives of Vincent Van Gogh to his brother, Theo. They are all good because they tell things in an unpretentious way—they just talk.

Next time you write a letter, even a business or formal letter to a superior, a client, or a stranger, make an effort to draw the reader into it, but remember, just talk. Appeal to him or her by mentioning something of great mutual concern. Weave a story—true or fabricated, depending on the reason for the letter—that will cause the reader's thumbs to sweat through the stationery. If you've ever received a letter from the head of, say, Covenant House for young runaways, or Hale House, where the late Mother Hale's work with AIDS and crack babies continues, you know what I mean. The concept of the compelling letter applies also to query letters to editors and letters to potential grantors (see Chapter 5, *On Grantwriting*).

Dr. Chopra's "Model" Letter to Little Ol' Me

Well, all right, I admit it says "Dear Friend," but I have a Gothic imagination. Even though it had been mailed to thousands of people, the letter made me feel I am in fact a friend of Dr. Deepak Chopra, an endocrinologist who has become one of the world's greatest mind/body teachers, philosophers, and practitioners. (He's now also a novelist.)

This brief excerpt of Chopra's letter gives you a straightforward but effective model for letters you want or have to write.

> Dear Friend,
>   As a health professional...I began asking myself, "Am I doing all I can for my patients? How can I better serve their needs?" ... (H)ealth is not merely the absence of disease but a state of harmony and well-being that permeates every cell of the body and every corner of the mind...
>   When I was asked to work with...the Sharp Institute for Human Potential and Mind Body Medicine, I...would finally be able to combine my training and experience in Western and mind body medicine. The training has been designed to be accessible to all health professionals...with an interest in...the therapeutic applications of mind body medicine and Ayurveda...

And so forth. Dr. Chopra concludes the letter by saying he will be conducting several sessions and how honored he is that distinguished experts will also be participating in the program. I guess I'm a fan, but I believe this is an informative, pleasant letter whose format and style we can use to our advantage.

The Interview as a Staple of Journal- and Feature-Writing

Having worked for many years as a daily newspaper reporter with deadlines coming at me like harpoons at a whale-hunt, I learned to love the interview. No matter what the topic, an interview with persons who know about the topic can enliven a story the way nothing else can.

The trick to the interview, as I see it, is to guide a person toward loosening up and giving you terrific quotes. Crack the initial, pleasant chit-chat to get hold of the nutmeat, the stuff your article needs. You don't have all day. If a person is dull, find someone else who will speak more engagingly. Or use the dull one's quotes for fundamental information on the topic, and then locate a renegade who will stir things up. Never forget to request an interview and permission to publish the interviewee's statements.

How to Extract the Best From an Interviewee

Use therapeutic communication techniques—open-ended questions, reflection, and so on—when doing an interview.

I discovered that my nurse's training helped me get wonderful material from even the most reticent people. Just as you would engage your client or patient in conversation, you can interview a doctor or therapist or whomever: How do you feel about...? What are the problems of...? Tell me more about... What would it take to...? Give me a mental picture of... Let the person talk, and have the good sense to know when the interview is over.

Listening Well Is the Key to a Good Interview

A major point of interviewing is to listen well and read signals. **Listen, listen, listen** to what your interviewee has to say. Notice the way he or she says it. Describing body language comes in handy. Be certain to ask the right questions of the right person.

For instance, it may not make sense to interview a physical therapist for an article pertaining to the newly expanded role of the nurse practitioner. When you have to drive a nail, you won't find a spoon of much help. The correct "tools" make all the difference.

Use a small tape recorder if you can't write fast or if you may not catch everything someone says. But beware of so-called high technology: Not only do some interviewees object to being taped, but malfunctions love to occur at crucial moments. This happened to me during an interview with Eileen Elias Freeman, who wrote *Touched By Angels*. The tape recorder that cost me nearly $200 refused to work. Although I took some notes on a reporter's pad, I was relying on the recorder. To top things off, I realized I had forgotten to put the film I bought in my camera case. I felt like Dopey the Dwarf, further intimidated by the fact that the article was to be published in *The New York Times*.

Ms. Freeman quickly offered her interpretation of what was happening: She said dark (bad) angels didn't want me to help spread her good word, and they were out to foil me.

"Let's make sure they fail," Ms. Freeman said, as she sent the friend who had accompanied me that day to a nearby store for film. And so it came to pass that the dark angels failed miserably; the story was one of my best, and Ms. Freeman was delighted.

Moral: You can survive anything with a few sharpened pencils, a notebook, and the courage to slow the interview down so you can take accurate notes. Don't be afraid to ask an interviewee to repeat, explain, or spell something. I remember reading an interview of a physician in which the reporter used the word "hypernia." She meant "hyperpnea," or rapid breathing, but she didn't think to ask the doctor about it, and, worst of all, she thought she knew how to spell it. And none of the editors caught the mistake or questioned the word. An accurate quote does far better than a foggy paraphrase.

Not Everyone Is Nice; Not Everyone Is Eloquent

Ask directly for the information you need for your article. Don't think you must know everything about a person's works or life before you can interview him or her. You cannot know everything. Ahead of time, make a list of intelligent questions you think are pertinent. Make sure you have a pen that functions and something more professional-looking than the back of a crinkled Citibank envelope to write on.

If you get flustered, laugh at yourself. Be patient; interviews are strange animals that, despite rotten strokes of luck, somehow land on their feet. Above all, don't be an icy interviewer.

Let the Interviewee Take the Floor

William Zinsser, author of *On Writing Well*, says: "His own words will always be better than yours, even if you are the most elegant stylist in the land... the inflection of his speaking voice and the idiosyncrasies of how he puts a sentence together. They contain the regionalisms of his conversation and the lingo of his trade. They convey his enthusiasms. This is a person talking to the reader directly, not through the filter of a writer. As soon as a writer steps in, everybody else's experience becomes secondhand."

Writing an Article for a Professional Journal

Professional journals come in all shapes and sizes. Some are keen on mainstream-type writing on topics of general interest, and some stick to esoteric, technical pieces. Some pay big bucks, some pay small amounts, say, $50 per published page, and others pay in contributors' copies. Most journals have staff writers but seek freelance pieces, too.

Freelance contributors have the best chance of getting published by offering editors well-written, unusual essays, how-to articles, and investigative reports with sidebars (those boxed-off, short pieces that pertain to the main article but offer tips, extra information, or another perspective).

Most specialized journals and magazines offer guidelines for writers at no charge. These guidelines will tell you what types of articles the publication needs, whom they wish to write them, and how they expect the manuscript to be constructed. Survey a publication by looking carefully at all the past year's issues in order to familiarize yourself with the magazine's style and approach. What topics did they cover? What's their stand on issues of the field? Do they favor a conversational style or a highly academic or technical style with bells, whistles, and footnotes?

Don't query a publication you've never laid eyes on—an editor spots this common faux pas like you'd spot a giraffe in your foyer. Request the guidelines, then query the editor about the idea you believe will "work" for the publication. (Many a rejection letter contains the phrase "It doesn't work for us at this time.")

Writing a Research Paper

Every college or university program requires students to do some form of research papers that "argue," though not in anger, a specific idea or topic. A very long version of the research paper is a thesis, which is discussed below. Shorter papers may range from 8 to 20 pages. Whatever the length, each paper should shed light on a topic and begin with a strong thesis statement.

Monmouth University, in West Long Branch, NJ, offers the following guidelines, which I have annotated in certain places, for effective written argumentation:

1. Compose a thesis or statement of topic to answer a question directly.

2. Develop a clear, logically organized argument.

3. Demonstrate accurate understanding of source material. (In other words, pick a topic you have some interest in and hunt for items written by others that emphasize or support your argument. Be careful of quoting material out of context.)

4. Define key terms where necessary. (Be careful of using jargon; you're better off to clarify technical terms. Moreover, don't assume that your reader is familiar with the key terms.)

5. Avoid irrelevant discussion. (Don't be afraid to include anecdotes or case studies that differ greatly from one another to illuminate the intricacies of a topic.)

6. Organize the argument in paragraphs; the average paragraph consists of five to eight sentences. (Try not to be so calculating about this, however. You need not add an eighth sentence unless the argument

requires it; on the other hand, you may need to make a paragraph nine or 10 sentences long if the extra sentences encourage and enhance the flow of your argument.)

7. Use paraphrase, summary, and quotation appropriately; include accurate parenthetical references to source material. (Paraphrasing means putting into your own words or in clarifying words what someone has said or written. This is distinct from quoting a spoken or written passage, which means using the words verbatim and indicating their source by quotation marks at the beginning and end. A summary, or condensation of the topic and the arguments, may use both paraphrasing and quotations as long as they are powerful and concise.)

8. Use appropriate language. (Please eliminate the unnecessary use of the word "like"—and the like—in formal writing unless you are quoting a teenager who'll say, "Like, I understand how she feels, but I'm like, what can I do about it?" You may find that taking out the "likes," "wells," and other superfluous words removes the authenticity of a person's speech pattern. As a rule, write the way you talk, but if you talk too colloquially, you may sound childish, strange, or inappropriate on paper unless you're trying to be the next J.D. Salinger.)

9. Compose sentences with enough variety to sustain the reader's interest and sufficient complexity to communicate the relationships between ideas.

10. Follow the rules of standard written English grammar, punctuation, and spelling. (This book is designed to help you do exactly that.)

The research paper, please remember, must contain research, which means offering the reader what experts in the field have to say about the topic you've chosen for your paper. Think about the topic: what is its nature, what do people already know about it, what don't they know, what controversies exist, what has recently been discovered, what point of view has been discarded because of newer ideas, etc.

When you choose a topic for a research paper, locate all the literature you can on that topic. Extract timely information, excellent quotes, and any material that supports your topic.

You need to create a thesis statement, an argument for or against it, and a reasonable conclusion. As I see it, a research paper should:

1.   Have a "reason for living," i.e., a strong point of view or important information.
2.   Have an enticing opening paragraph; as Jacques Barzun put it in his book *Simple & Direct: A Rhetoric for Writers*, "Readers are shy birds that have to be coaxed to come nearer." Some of those birds are your professors and your peers who are to read and evaluate your work.
3.   Pose a question or describe a problem and resolve it (or at least offer a semblance of a resolution).
4.   Use the most powerful quotes from experts on the topic.
5.   Properly identify people and situations for the reader, e.g., Dr. Bella J. May, professor of physical therapy at the University of Georgia.
6.   Have an inherent sense of excitement, experimentation, or fun with the topic, as opposed to reiterating an old, well-known point of view; original thinking is the stuff of history.
7.   Be well-groomed, i.e., clean paper; clear letters; a cover sheet for the title, by-line, name of the course, instructor's name and date; a consistent style (such as Turabian or whatever the course or college requires); a bibliography that is updated and easy to read; italics where necessary for clarity and emphasis; and the overall look of a professional job.
8.   Be handed in on time.
9.   Not be a recycled version of your older sister's paper.
10. Not be a paper pilfered or written by someone else.

As a health professional, you need to communicate often, frequently at length and in your own words. Rarely will you be in a test-like situation, in which you have a multiple choice format or brief essay questions to answer.

Life is a story, not a quiz. Health care is drama, intricately stitched tapestries that represent each client's unique life, not a fill-in-the-blanks standard form.

I urge you to take a bit more kindly to research papers. Oh, sure, they can be as much fun to do as defrosting your refrigerator, especially when you're putting in long hours on the job. You don't have to like research papers, but you'll do yourself a favor by writing simply and directly about a topic close to your heart. And to the victor go the spoils—research papers are vital exercises that can even improve your style of caregiving.

Writing a Thesis

First you need to understand and develop a thesis statement. This is applicable to any kind of writing, but especially to the thesis required of some baccalaureate and graduate degree programs. In his book, *Writing Voyage*, Thomas Tyner suggests the following points:

- A thesis statement expresses the main idea you want to develop in a paper. It usually expresses your viewpoint on the topic.
- Your thesis statement determines the way in which you develop a topic in a paper. You write your paper in support of your thesis.
- A thesis is to an essay what a topic sentence is to a paragraph; it expresses the main idea. Just as the sentences within the paragraph relate to the topic sentence, the paragraphs within a paper relate to the thesis statement.
- Without a thesis, a paper lacks direction. There is no controlling idea to tie the paragraphs together and to help the reader understand the writer's intent.
- There is no "right" or "wrong" thesis statement; it reflects the way a writer views a particular topic. The effectiveness of the thesis is usually determined by how well it is supported in the paper.

Tyner gives examples of topics and theses, such as:

Topic: Alcoholism.

Thesis: Teenage alcoholism is a more serious problem than drug use.

Thesis: Alcoholism is increasingly becoming a woman's disease.

Thesis: Alcoholism is an overrated health problem in America.

With the concept of the thesis statement firmly implanted, you can go on to write an entire essay called a thesis in academic circles. Although universities differ in their requirements for a thesis, most often it is an analytical or argumentative essay based on original research that substantiates a particular point of view.

The components of an academic thesis usually include an abstract, or a summary of the thesis statement and the intent of the writer; the informative, argumentative, persuasive, or analytical body of the thesis; conclusion; footnotes; and bibliography. Theses may be as short as 30 pages or as long as the advisor requests. Both student and academic advisor must be clear on what the thesis is to contain and accomplish. Frequently, an advisor must approve the thesis statement beforehand, and the school adopts a certain style format to which you must adhere. I believe writing on a fresh topic or having a fresh approach to an old one supersedes which style you use. A thesis merely reiterates what everyone else already knows about a topic, while an inventive thesis makes a valuable contribution to your profession.

Jacques Barzun in his book, *Simple & Direct*, writes: "In a thesis or argument, think of the objections you must forestall, framing and answering them. In a didactic piece, think of the confusions and errors you must remove to make the teaching clear. In a description, think of the unknowns that must be depicted before the whole can be rightly imagined. With a slight effort of the kind at the start—a challenge to utterance—you will find your pretense disappearing and a real concern creeping in."

Other considerations for writing a thesis are well-delineated in *Patterns for College Writing*, by Laurie G. Kirszner, of the Philadelphia College of Pharmacy and Science, and Stephen R. Mandell, of Drexel University. These authors advocate many approaches to the thesis- or essay-writing process, from understanding the assignment to actual writing structure. They emphasize narration, description, exemplification, process (e.g., a process essay on how something is done), cause and effect, comparison and contrast, classification and division, definition and argumentation, all tools to help you get started and to satisfactorily complete your thesis.

My 30-page baccalaureate thesis worked out well as a photo-essay of a building designed by architect Stanford White, substantiated by original and secondary research on White and the visionary Stewart Hartshorn of Short Hills, NJ. Using APA style (see Chapter 8, *On Style*), I described the building in great detail—which parts were originally White's design and which parts had been redone, mutilated, or eliminated. I never sought publication, but the thesis is in a local library. It's nice to know your research is welcomed by the community and other researchers and thesis writers, so you may wish to offer your thesis to a library collection.

Writing for a Newsletter or House Organ

This, my friends, is conversational writing whose purpose is to inform, entertain, and promote employee morale of a corporation or organization, or a group of people with the same interests, such as the "AngelWatch" newsletter put out by Eileen Freeman for angel-watchers and devotees, or newsletters put out by organizations such as the National Association of Home Care (NAHC). Interviews, features on company events, profiles of individuals or programs, etc., work very well.

Good photographs help enormously, although I must say most newsletters I've seen lean toward the "rack 'em and stack 'em" line-up photos, and what I derogatorily refer to as "yearbook pictures." I prefer to see well-composed pictures of people on the job or doing something other than just flashing their teeth for the camera. Active photos, like active writing, provide eye-catching page layouts that attract readers. The newsletter should represent the organization with dignity and reality. Even the Mickey Mouse Club goes for dignity and reality. The best writing style for newsletters, I believe, emulates good reports and features of the daily newspaper.

Writing a News Release

A news release is a nuts-and-bolts version of a news report. Nuts-and-bolts answer the questions Who, What, When, Where, How, and Why as concisely as possible. Written in an informal but well-mannered style, good reports separate fact from opinion and steer clear of excessive details. The best news releases are fairly short and arrive on an editor's desk in a "press kit."

The press kit contains everything an editor needs to plunk the story into a waiting "news hole," or space in the publication. The components of a press kit are:

1.   The news release
2.   Pertinent photographs (or slides) with clear identification on the back or on tags attached to each photo
3.   Background information on the topic or subject, such as resumes, published clippings or reviews, brochures, books, etc.
4.   Name and telephone number of the contact person, and times he or she may be reached

The American Medical Association provided this "Media Alert." Sent on AMA stationery, it is an excellent example of a news release:

> SUNDAY, OCTOBER 1, 1995
> WHO WILL MAKE DECISIONS ABOUT YOUR HEALTH CARE IF YOU'RE UNABLE TO DO SO?
> Survey finds more than one-half of Americans know little or nothing about health care advance directives.
> MIAMI BEACH—More than two-thirds of Americans do not have "living wills," although almost three-fourths say the document is important, according to a report released today by the American Medical Association (AMA).
>   The report, which details results of a survey conducted by the AMA, reveals that the nation is wholly unfamiliar with health care advance directives, despite education campaigns and federal laws calling for their use. An advance directive is a document in which you give instructions about your health care if, in the future, you cannot speak for yourself.

In response to the report, the AMA, the American Association of Retired Persons (AARP), and the American Bar Association (ABA) today released "Shaping Your Health Care Future with Health Care Advance Directives," a patient guide that combines a living will and health care power of attorney into a single, comprehensive document. According to the report, the pressure on the patient's family to make health care choices can be overwhelming in cases where there has been no prior conversation about the patient's wishes. "Family members suffer great angst over determining what their ill family member would have wanted. Decisions can be tempered by fear of personal loss if the sick person dies or a sense of relief if the stress of caring for the sick person has been overbearing," states the report.

"Each American adult must protect themselves and take the necessary precautions so they are in control of their health care decisions," said P. John Seward, MD, chair, AMA Board of Trustees. "The advance directive form we've created can be used nationwide. It'll give patients and their families peace of mind and can help relieve family stress."

According to the report, the opportunity to express wishes about end-of-life care is a significant means of alleviating public anxieties surrounding death in the modern age. Technological advance has resulted in prolonged life, but the care may be of marginal value, depending on the patients' assessment of their quality of life. Completing an advance directive can give individuals confidence that they will maintain control of their end-of-life treatment and will be provided care commensurate with their wishes.

"Preparing an advance directive now is a way to make sure your voice is heard if you should become unable to make your own decisions about medical care," said AARP Board Member Marie Sonderman, RN. "It's a wise investment for yourself and one of the most valuable gifts you can give to those close to you."

The advance directive form found in the AMA, ABA, AARP booklet is designed to be portable, meeting most state law requirements. In the few states with unusual enforcement requirements, health care providers still must follow the principle of adhering to a patient's wishes. The three organizations are urging all states to recognize a national model, such as the advance directive form found in the booklet.

"The joint authorship of this booklet by the AMA, ABA, and the AARP should eliminate confusion about what the law on advance directives is and how to handle issues surrounding terminal illness," said Roberta Cooper Ramo, president, ABA.

Founded in 1847, the AMA is a voluntary membership organization of physicians and medical students and the world's largest publisher of scientific and medical information. The AARP is the nation's leading organization for people age 50 and older. As the national voice for the legal profession, the ABA has initiated hundreds of programs addressing a wide range of public concerns, from child abuse and domestic violence to the law-related concerns of elder persons.

For a review copy of "Shaping Your Health Care Future with Health Care Advance Directives," contact the AMA's Department of News & Information at 312-464-4430.

If you are responsible for alerting the media of your organization's events, progress, or prominent personalities, you can use this release as a model.

Writing In-Service Workshop Handouts

Workshop materials typically are photocopied sheets of paper, perhaps with looseleaf holes and placed in a notebook.

Here again, the writing style is concise, with large, boldface headings and, if possible, a graphic or illustration that enhances the topic. Outlines and lists highlighting the workshop agenda are also acceptable as hand-outs; excerpts from pertinent literature may be copied and distributed to the group. Handouts serve as reminders and reinforcements of the material covered in the workshop or in-service, so avoid inundating participants with paper. Give them only the essentials. They can take notes on something esoteric or of particular interest to them.

Charting and Other Documentation

Charts and forms filled out on the job are usually handwritten. Make a great effort to write legibly. Legible documents avoid confusion among staff and protect both the one who writes and the next one who reads it. In charting, tell **what you observed**. You are free to use abbreviations and jargon appropriate to your field.

Charts are not the place to ventilate anger or other emotion, however, nor are they the vehicle for sarcasm and bias. The team meeting or consultations among professionals provides time for the expression of personal ideas or problems. Don't forget to sign your name on the chart: It is perhaps your most important "by-line."

Writing a Book

Ah, there's the rub! Now we can really hit the grid of writers' agonies, ecstasies, blah periods, and numb periods, because the book, usually the longest piece of writing, gives you plenty of time for all of that. My first bit of advice for the aspiring author is: Step One—Get published in journals, newspapers, and magazines before you try a book. That way you develop your interests and expertise, become familiar with the publishing process, and learn who your audience is. Step Two—Write a proposal for a book. Once you have a few impressive clippings, you are better equipped to write a book proposal that will attract an agent. Here are guidelines for writing a proposal:

1. Title page: The title of the book, the author's name, and the agent's name.
2. Introduction: An overview of the book and the author's credentials.

    The Overview—Seize the eye and interest of a busy editor with a compelling or funny anecdote, quote, or event. Tell what the book is about briefly and why people will want to read it. Keep the style conversational; use the same tone as if you were writing a letter to a dear friend.

    About the Author(s)—Who are you and why are you writing this book?

3.   Chapter descriptions: Give a full or partial page of prose describing each chapter, but make your text continuous. Don't start a new page for each chapter or your proposal will look choppy. Describe the chapter, not the subject matter, and give each chapter a structure: "The chapter opens with..." Show the editor you've put together a book with a logical sequence of ideas or events. Again, an eye-catching, pithy header or a quote may enhance each chapter. You can divide the book into large sections, each section containing several chapters, or you can have many small sections, depending upon your subject and style. No matter what, organize the book well.

4.   Sample chapter: This chapter is the one you most want to write. Do a marvelous job, because this will give the editor the best impression of the book and how you will handle it. If you have a knack for writing humorous prose, use it here.

5.   Tell an editor about other parts of the book—front- and backmatter, such as a foreword (often written by a well-known person or authority), introduction, quotes for the book, photographs or illustrations, etc. Give an approximate length in book pages. Specify how much time you need to write the book. It is also important to specify how your book competes with others on the same subject—more in-depth material, a different or improved approach to the subject, etc. Identify other books on the market and tell why yours is more attractive.

6.   Attach newspaper or magazine articles written by you. Good reviews or comments about your work always help. If the articles are long, underline in pen or bracket on the side the most important parts. Don't use a highlighter. It photocopies black, covering up the line of type. Include a list of other books or articles you have published, and anything you think will help.

Poetry as Therapy

Most professional writers' first writings were poems. Young people's poems, particularly adolescents' poems, often reveal, exonerate, and validate an angry, self-searching time.

Susan Dion's booklet *Write Now* touts poetry as a flow of thought that can foster your creative spirit and blow off steam whether you are the patient or the caregiver.

Dion encourages us to: "Experiment. Try different styles and many subjects... Don't worry about style or form initially (unless you prefer the challenge of rigid form)...Use childhood memories...old mementos or photographs...Write short poems at various times of the week...to capture the essence of how you feel or think in that moment...Try some poems focusing on common items: a pair of socks thrown on the floor...a frayed rug...a bowl of morning cereal...Funny, crazy poems can be a real release... such as all the reasons I'm annoyed by_____ or the silliness of being ill and confined."

Chapter 5
On Grantwriting
Margaret M. Lundrigan, MSW, LCSW

Grantwriting

I turned this segment of the book over to Margaret M. Lundrigan, MSW, LCSW, who has a stronger stomach than I for discussing grants. Margaret and I were both hired by a Visiting Nurse Association as supervisors of grant research. Neither of us had any grantwriting experience, but we plunged in and managed to acquire more than $300,000 for the company in about a year and a half.

The Nature of the Beast

There is no middle-of-the-road opinion on grants. For some, grants hold the lure of pirate treasure, with the aura of the Irish sweepstakes thrown in. For others it is as mysterious as the esoteric brotherhoods, or as exciting as filling out an expense report. For others—root canal. Where does the truth lie? Probably in a swirling conglomeration of all the above. Every agency has a senior administrator who can tell you about the grant that saved the agency from certain destruction, the grant that got away (because the competition had an in with the funders), and the grant that made that nincompoop Shirley a senior vice president/company darling. Who knew she could write anything more than her name?

The Reason for Grants

Professionals in the human service fields need to have at least a rudimentary knowledge of foundation-giving and the grant-proposal process, because grants have become one of the mechanisms that affects an organization's economic health, including individual jobs. Balk as we may, grants do represent a real effort to achieve fairness and equity in the distribution of funds. There are limited resources and innumerable causes or needs. Rather than arbitrarily deciding which organizations or programs should receive financial assistance and how much they should receive, government agencies and philanthropic foundations make it known that they have funds available and are interested in providing funds for certain types of programs.

These agencies and foundations set criteria that must be met if funding is to be awarded. In essence, the function of a foundation or donor is that of an administrative body responsible for overseeing and dispensing funds allocated for a particular cause, e.g., the education of disadvantaged children.

More Reasons to Be Kind to Grants

Many grantors intend to give a worthy project the resources to start up—seed money. The grantors then suppose that once the project is operational, the grantees will be able to acquire funding to keep it going. If funding does not continue, grantors may decide the project was not as worthy as they thought or that the grantees did not put sufficient effort into obtaining money from other sources. Health professionals seeking grant money must understand that if foundations continually supported the same projects, however worthwhile, the number of projects would be greatly reduced.

On the other hand, there are foundations formed expressly for the purpose of funding or identifying funding sources for certain projects or programs.

Matchmaker, Matchmaker, Make Me a Match

No grant, no matter how well-written or how deserving the cause, is worth the paper it is written on unless you send it to the appropriate funder. Some company foundations, such as Kellogg (the corn-flake people), prefer to support grass-roots programs, while others, such as Ben & Jerry's (ice cream products), gravitate toward smaller, more offbeat projects. The two bibles for grant-seekers are the *Foundation Grants Index 1997* and the *1997 Guide to Federal Funding for Governments and Non-Profits*, both comprehensive sources, among others, of public and private funders.

The *Foundation Grants Index 1997*, published by the Foundation Center of New York, contains clear, concise information on nearly all private foundations in existence. The information includes the foundation's philosophy of giving, target populations, amounts of grants, application procedures, and when grants are reviewed. Written in fine print and a legalese format, the *1997 Guide to Federal Funding for Governments and Non-Profits* makes *Beowulf* seem like a day in the park. Don't despair, however: There are ways around this difficult situation other than putting an attorney on retainer. Books on how to write successful grants, particularly addressing the issue of matching the "right" funder with the "right" program, are available in the library and bookstores.

Big Foundation, Big Money?

Not necessarily so! The temptation to submit grant proposals to large, attractive, wealthy foundations may be hard to resist. When we read of foundations whose gifts fall generally into the six-figure range, somehow we feel if they really understood what we are trying to do, they surely would beat a path to our door with checkbook in hand. But foundations are sophisticated consumers, and they mean what they say. If they are in the business of helping teenage substance abusers, it is unlikely they will help middle-aged substance abusers.

Groundwork for Grants

The first rule of grantwriting is to clearly identify your goals and objectives. If you can't specify what you want to achieve, your chances of success are nil. For example, the goal of achieving peace on Earth is admirable, but it is probably not a fundable project. If you want to send 20 students to a 6-month seminar on conflict resolution, you may well have a fundable project. After you determine that your project can be carried out, you must define criteria for selecting the students, devise a realistic budget including the precise cost per student, consider the efficacy of the seminar, and describe some plan to continue funding of this project after the initial grant runs out.

Elements of a Grant Proposal

Grant proposals provide answers to the questions Who (or what client population), Why (what need is being addressed), How (the method of help), When (duration of the project), How Much (itemized budget outlining the costs of developing and delivering the services), and—that awful question—How We Will Go On Without You (plans for supporting the project after the grant period). The following are typical elements you must illuminate.

Covering, or Cover, Letter

A business letter tops the package and goes to the foundation or company grant officer or contact person. So many cover letters are stiff and full of clichés! I say get real. Introduce your agency or program, offer a nutshell description of your project and its significance, and leave the rest of the work to your proposal.

Summary

The summary, a synopsis of the information contained in the grant proposal, concisely presents what the project is and what you expect to accomplish. Many grantors' standard proposal forms provide a separate sheet and limited space in which to write the summary, possibly the hardest part of the proposal to write. Give the summary full steam. A thumbnail sketch of the entire project, the summary is extremely important and the most scrutinized of the components, except perhaps the budget. If the summary fails to entice the reader, the body of the grant won't entice the reader.

Introduction

The introduction is a kind of resume of your agency or organization. Generally, this section contains the organization's mission statement, why the organization was founded, its goals, and history of success. Although most agencies have a mission statement as a main part of their literature, some do not have a formal, prepared statement.

Grantwriters may be taken aback to discover that no one has formally stated why the agency came to be. The introduction establishes the agency's credentials to perform the services proposed in the grant application. Letters of support from other agencies and individuals who know the agency's work enhance the credibility of the agency.

Problem Statement

This is the rationale for funding the project. Also called a needs assessment, the problem statement documents a problem calling for a program to be developed by an agency. When an agency devises and prepares to operate a program for the resolution of the problem, oftentimes the program deserves to be funded. For instance, a mobile outreach clinic program is designed by nurses to deal with the increase of homeless people who do not have access to medical care. It is important to be specific: "There has been a 30% increase in the number of homeless persons in River City, many of them the deinstitutionalized mentally ill who have no access to the health care delivery system." Official census records and conducting a survey in a community may be used to help document needs.

The problem statement also offers the best vehicle for making an emotional appeal to a potential funder. Jerry Lewis knows this very well. His telethons jump on people's heartstrings to loosen their pursestrings. When Jerry, Jerry's Kids, and the guest celebrities are through, there isn't a dry eye in the house. The millions of dollars donated to muscular dystrophy organizations as a result of the annual telethon bespeak its enormous success.

In your problem statement, include anecdotes—true stories about people in great need and what happened to

them because of grant money or because of the lack of it—
that imbue a personal flavor to the kind of care given by an
agency. Anecdotes are the heart and soul of the grant
proposal: If they are not compelling and do not speak to
humanity and compassion, the most beautifully formulated
program will not seem valuable to a funder. When the
anecdotes are bolstered by well-documented need, they
create a grant's "reason for living."

Objectives

This section describes what is to be achieved in
measurable terms. An organization's goal may be to
improve the literacy rate for a group of low-income
students. A measurable objective might be to increase by 1
year the average reading level of 10th-grade students.
Objectives should not be confused with methods. The
objective specifies what is to be accomplished. While goals
may be general, objectives need to be specific and
quantifiable.

Methods

Here you give the nuts and bolts of how you intend to
operate the program to be funded. This section details the
activities that will occur in the program. For example, you
are proposing a program to inoculate 200 school children
against the Hepatitis B virus. How is this going to happen?
Will you employ a nurse or physician to inoculate the
children? Will the designated health professional go to a
school or community organization, or will the children be
transported to the professional's workplace? If so, how will
transportation be provided? How will the children be
selected? How will the vaccine be acquired? How will all
permissions be obtained? The answers to these questions
define your method of operation.

Evaluation

Criteria for determining if goals and objectives have
been accomplished are an important component in your
grant proposal. A funder wants to know his or her money is

well spent and the program deserving. Usually you tell funders the program will be scrutinized relentlessly by gimlet eyes throughout the program, and problem areas will be continuously adjusted as necessary. That's the truth, right? Always be truthful.

Budget

This is an itemized account of how the requested funds will be spent, down to the penny, if possible. Whether in the form of a line budget (i.e., a listing of services, employees, etc. on the left and costs in dollars lined up with them to the right) or a budget narrative (paragraphs describing costs and how they will be allocated), the budget is a numerical reflection of the money you need in order to deliver your services. If you are not an accountant or responsible for preparing a budget, enlist the aid of a knowledgeable person. Most health care agencies and organizations employ persons with financial acumen and designate certain ones to work with grantwriters. The quality of the budget is crucial information to both your agency and the funder. Budgets should never be padded or underestimated; either extreme may have a negative impact on the grant's viability.

Future Funding

Now for a nasty question: How will your agency obtain funds for a previously funded program after the initial grant money is gone? With the exception of programs typically funded through legislation on a long-term basis, many grants, particularly those of private foundations, are granted with the understanding that there are definite plans for the program to become self-sustaining.

There are any number of ways in which a program can become self-supporting, from charging for the service, to fund-raising, to appealing to local benefactors. Whatever route you choose, it has to be credible.

Special Effects

In an effort to make their grants stand out, many writers resort to high-powered Madison Avenue sell techniques such as videos, flow charts, and expensive bindings. To my mind and from my experience, there is one rule about this sort of thing: **don't**. Although you may feel you are in the running for the social service academy awards, the grantor will probably have two questions: Who paid for all this flashy stuff? Is this how our money will be spent? In an era in which the spending habits of many philanthropic organizations are being looked at, these tactics raise a red flag in the funders' minds. The funders are more likely to be impressed by a proposal that is reader-friendly and follows the guidelines.

The Good Thing About Rejection

A rejected grant proposal can arouse more hostility than 20 years of psychotherapy. The rejection follows Dr. Elisabeth Kübler-Ross' stages of grief over impending death or after a major trauma:

1.   Denial, or It can't be! They must have mixed us up with someone else! They're kidding!
2.   Anger, or Those monsters! I hope their yacht springs a leak in shark-infested waters! I hope they're drummed out of the Daughters of the American Revolution because of Grandmama's indiscretion aboard the Mayflower.
3.   Bargaining, or If I rewrite the proposal, surely they will reconsider, or if I call them and...
4.   Depression, or I might as well give up grantwriting and kill myself with a rock.
5.   Acceptance, or They rejected our proposal not because it lacked merit, but because they were looking for a collaborative effort. Let's get some valuable feedback from them, and start working on another proposal.

Say Thank You to the Nice Man

When the funders come through and send that fabulous letter saying yes, communicate your gratitude immediately and find out what the next step is in the funding process.

Grantspeak

Private foundation: An organization formed for the purpose of providing assistance to individuals and groups engaged in an activity of particular interest.

Operating foundation: An organization that exists to engage funding for a specific organization, such as museums and hospitals. Do not apply to them for grants. They fund themselves.

In-kind contribution: Help given not in the form of money, but in the form of equipment, expertise, or other items, such as office space or services.

Guidelines: The requirements that must be met in order to be considered for a grant.

Proposal: A written request, usually involving a set of standard forms sent by the potential funder, for funding for a project or program.

Seed money: Money funded to start a project or program.

Operating grant: A grant that pays for the day-to-day operating expenses of an organization. These may be the most difficult grants to obtain.

Matching funds: A requirement that equal funds be contributed to the project by the parent organization. Some large companies will match their employees' contributions to charitable organizations.

RFP: Request for Proposal, an announcement made by a funder indicating the availability of funds or grants for specific activities. The RFP also states the guidelines or criteria that must be met for consideration.

Trustee: An officer or board member of an organization who plays a decision-making role in the allocations of a foundation's grants.

Section 501(3)(c): A section of the Internal Revenue Service (IRS) code that qualifies non-profit organizations to be tax-exempt.

Form 990-PF: A form required by law of all foundations to submit to the IRS. These forms contain financial information regarding the foundation.

General Rules for Grantwriters

- Research to find the best match of your program's needs and the funders' interests or requirements.
- Use the writing process to clarify. The grantwriting process can expose program weaknesses and inconsistencies.
- Use rejection as a learning process. Maintain contact with funders. Thank them for their consideration. Request feedback, especially if you plan to apply for a grant from the same funder next year.
- Network with colleagues to find new sources of grant money. Share the knowledge you have with others.
- Take a grantwriting course. Courses are given by a number of organizations, including The Foundation Center in New York City, The Grantsmanship Center, and some private organizations. These courses run from a few hours to as long as a week. Even the short ones can quickly run you through the mechanics of the grantwriting process and give you some confidence. Many agencies or other employers are willing to pay for your tuition and expenses.
- Throw back the small fish. Some funders provide only small amounts of assistance, are extremely picky, and waste a lot of your time.

Chapter 6
On Grammar

Why Didn't I Pay Closer Attention in Grammar School?

Grammar scares people. Grammar has scared so many people that today's elementary-school teachers may avoid teaching their students to diagram sentences or master inflection and syntax (basically, sentence structure). The intensive study of and respect for grammar may have already gone the way of Victorian diction lessons.

I advise health professionals to brush up on at least the major points of English grammar. After all, you can never look too good in print.

Thinking in Sentences

"We think in sentences, and the way we think is the way we see. If we think in the structure subject/verb/direct object, then that is how we form our world. By cracking open that syntax, we release energy and are able to see the world afresh and form a new angle."—Natalie Goldberg, *Writing Down the Bones.*

Grammar Offers a System of Writing

I owe much of my writing ability and desire to write to the fact that my grammar-school teachers actually taught grammar. In fifth grade, we diagrammed sentences till our little fingers ached. We learned the parts of speech: nouns, verbs, pronouns, adjectives, adverbs, interjections, conjunctions, prepositions, articles, and demonstratives. We were drilled on the parts of a sentence: subjects, verbs, objects, complements, and adverbials. And, through diagramming, we mulled over prepositional, appositive, participial, infinitive, gerund, and absolute phrases and endured adjective, adverb, and noun clauses on the brain as we slept.

In sum, the rules of grammar afforded me and my classmates a strong foundation in language arts, and therefore, in competent writing.

The Bare-Bones Approach to Grammar

I don't want any snoring during this section, so I'll address very concisely everything you always wanted to know about grammar but were afraid to ask. If you want to skip around in this section, particularly to home in on information you need pronto, that's fine with me. I recommend scanning most literature before deciding to read straight through, because I believe in synchronicity: You'll turn to the page that has on it exactly what means the most to you, what you should know, at any given moment. Try it.

Nouns: Boy, dog, sandwich are common, singular nouns; boys, dogs, sandwiches are plural nouns; Mickey Mouse, Arizona, Erickson, Bright's disease are proper nouns (names); patience, harmony, indulgence are abstract common nouns; lentils, wine, parsley are concrete common nouns; food, medicine are collective nouns.

Pronouns: I, we, you, he, she, it, they are subjective personal pronouns; me, us, you, him, her, it, them are objective personal pronouns; mine, yours, ours, his, hers, theirs are possessive pronouns, along with the determiner forms of possessive pronouns: my, our, your, his, her, its, their; myself, ourselves, themselves, yourself, yourselves, himself, herself, oneself, itself are reflexive pronouns; most, everybody, both, each, all, everything, everywhere, someone, somebody, any, anyone, neither, none, few, either, much, several, enough are indefinite pronouns; who, whom, whose, whoever, whomever are personal relative pronouns; which, whose, whichever, whatever are nonpersonal relative pronouns; that is a general pronoun.

The Subjective Case

Subjects in a sentence require the use of common nouns, proper nouns (names), and subjective personal pronouns: "she and I," "he and his colleagues," "Mr. and Mrs. Claus," "Nancy and her fellow patients," "the OT," "a dietitian," etc.

Never write, "Her and me went to the client's home" or "Him and the doctor talked in the hallway." Him, her, and me are only for objective use. (See The Objective Case.) *Correct:* "She and I went...," "He and the doctor talked... "

Noun-Verb, or Subject-Verb, Agreement

Nouns and verbs—the action words—must agree. For example, "Martha don't like you," is wrong. *Correct:* "Martha (noun/subject) does not (verb) like you." Or, "The data creates a dilemma" is wrong. *Correct:* "The data (plural noun/subject) create (verb) a dilemma." BUT, "Statistics is a course most graduate students dread." "Controlled dangerous substances is a subject of great concern in home health care."

If you invert the sentence you can often determine the subject of the sentence better, e.g., "A subject of great concern in home health care is controlled dangerous substances."

Once you know what the subject is, you can decide on the proper verb. Also remember that more than one subject requires a plural form of the verb, e.g., "The occupational therapist and the psychiatrist are planning a staff meeting." Or, "In the supply closet are a Foley catheter and a box of syringes."

Sentence Fragments

If there is no verb or no subject to form a complete sentence, you have a sentence fragment. A phrase beginning with if, since, so that, when, whether, whose, why, because, although, after, etc. may lead to an ungrammatical sentence fragment. In Diana Hacker's *The Bedford Handbook for Writers* some unacceptable sentence fragments are: "I had pushed these fears into one of those quiet places in my mind. Hoping they would stay there asleep," and "To give my family a comfortable, secure home life. That is my most important goal."

The Acceptable Sentence Fragment

Sometimes writers use sentence fragments for emphasis, as an element of style, to save words, or to answer a question. For example, *The Bedford Handbook for Writers* cites the following passage from *Hunger of Memory*, by Richard Rodriguez: "Following the dramatic Americanization of their children, even my parents grew more publicly confident. Especially my mother. She learned the names of all the people on our block."

Bedford adds this example: "Are these new drug tests 100% reliable? Not in the opinion of most experts."

In spoken English, we use many sentence fragments. In written English, use only those that add flavor, depth, and reader-friendliness to your piece.

Use Nouns Instead of Broad References

Clarify pronouns or antecedents (words that precede pronouns or broad references) by substituting nouns. An example is: "The rise of domestic violence in our country brought about the need for women's shelters. Health professionals recognize this (broad reference), but how do they reach out to the community to solve it?" Change the sentence to: "Health professionals recognize the problem..." Who and that, which and whose. Don't write "I know a patient that recovered very well from the accident." Write: "I know a patient who recovered..." A person is a who, whom, or whose; an inanimate object, an animal, or an idea is a that or which (unless you are writing about my dog, Francis, who is decidedly a who.)

Don't write, "My client lives with her seven children, three of which are therapists." Write: "My client lives with her seven children, three of whom are therapists."

The Objective Case

All too often I hear people use the subjective case instead of the objective, because, for some strange reason, they think the objective case sounds either unrefined or wrong. *Example:* "The therapist reported to she and I." OUCH! *Correct:* "The therapist reported to her and me." Would you say "Give the ball to I"? No. The correct form is objective: "Give the ball to me."

Would you say "The therapist went to the hospital with my family and I"? No. You would not say "with I." *Correct:* "The therapist went to the hospital with my family and me." *Incorrect:* The client expected the therapist and I to cure him. *Correct:* The client expected the therapist and me to cure him. (You would not say "He expected I.")

The word "between" uses the objective case, too: "Between you and me, the request is unrealistic." NOT "Between you and I." *Incorrect:* The competition grew between she and I. *Correct:* The competition grew between her and me.

The use of "better than" takes both subject and object, but the meaning of the sentence may change. Bedford gives this example: My husband likes football better than I (subjective). My husband likes football better than me (objective).

If you finish each sentence mentally, the first sentence means: My husband likes football better than I (do). But the second sentence means: My husband likes football better than (he likes) me.

The Possessive Case

To modify a gerund, i.e., a word that ends in -ing that functions as a noun, use the possessive case (my, our, your, his/her/its, their). *Incorrect:* The supervisor tolerates us coming in late on Fridays. *Correct:* The supervisor tolerates our coming in late on Fridays. *Incorrect:* Nurses tend to tolerate Dr. Smith coming in late. *Correct:* Nurses tend to tolerate Dr. Smith's coming in late.

Double Negatives

Avoid using "can't hardly," "can't barely," "won't never," etc. Double negatives may change the meaning to an undesired positive, such as, "She is not doing nothing," which actually means she is doing something. Notice the ungrammatical use of double negatives in the following examples: *Incorrect:* The manager is not doing nothing about poor scheduling. *Correct:* The manager is not doing anything about poor scheduling. *Incorrect:* They don't want no trouble. *Correct:* They don't want any trouble.

The use of double negatives may be acceptable, however, for emphasis, or when a positive meaning is intended. For example, "The health care team was not unhappy with its sense of camaraderie," which means the team was satisfied, though perhaps not delighted, with its sense of camaraderie. One of poet Maya Angelou's books, *Wouldn't Take Nothing for My Journey Now*, uses an acceptable double negative because of its style and emphasis.

A cartoon that appears in Marcia Lerner's *The Princeton Review Writing Smart* pokes fun at double negatives in songs: "Miss Ilene Kranshaw sings 100% Grammatically Correct Popular Tunes, featuring: 'You Aren't Anything But a Hound Dog,' 'It Doesn't Mean a Thing If It Hasn't Got That Swing,' and 'I'm Not Misbehaving.'" Sometimes there just ain't nothing like a good double negative.

Use Proper Verb Forms

Incorrect: I should have went to the pharmacy earlier. *Correct:* I should have gone to the pharmacy earlier.

Incorrect: The patient was woken up at midnight. *Correct:* The patient was awakened at midnight.

Incorrect: The children snuck out of the pediatric ward. *Correct:* The children sneaked out of the pediatric ward.

Incorrect: She might have saw a different person. *Correct:* She might have seen a different person.

Incorrect: I could have ate the whole thing. *Correct:* I could have eaten the whole thing.

Incorrect: Her mother brang her some flowers. *Correct:* Her mother brought her some flowers.

Incorrect: The therapist should have knew what to do. *Correct:* The therapist should have known what to do.

Incorrect: I was hurted, so I runned to the hospital. *Correct:* I was hurt, so I ran to the hospital.

Incorrect: Chemotherapy made the patient look all wore out. *Correct:* Chemotherapy made the patient look all worn out.

Incorrect: The criminal was hung at high noon. *Correct:* The criminal was hanged at high noon.

Incorrect: The IV line had broke. *Correct:* The IV line had broken.

Incorrect: The client had been beat up by her spouse. *Correct:* The client had been beaten up by her spouse.

Incorrect: I should have stood in bed. *Correct:* I should have stayed in bed.

Incorrect: He had drank too much. *Correct:* He had drunk too much.

Incorrect: A nurse had wrote the patient's will. *Correct:* A nurse had written the patient's will.

Incorrect: Miriam swum across the lake and drownded. *Correct:* Miriam swam across the lake and drowned.

Incorrect: The nutritionist hanged the vitamin chart on the wall. *Correct:* The nutritionist hung the vitamin chart on the wall.

Incorrect: After I run two miles, I lay down for a nap.
Correct: After I run two miles, I lie down for a nap.

Incorrect: Physical therapists are use to hard work.
Correct: Physical therapists are used to hard work.

Incorrect: The moon revolved around the earth. *Correct:*
The moon revolves around the earth.

Incorrect: If I was you, I'd leave tomorrow. *Correct:* If I
were you, I'd leave tomorrow.

Now you have an overview of the grammar mystique. I
suggest you refer to your style book if you run into trouble
with a word form or sentence structure, because with things
grammatical, one never knows, do one?

Chapter 7
On Punctuation

The "Road Signs" of Written Language

Punctuation marks tell the reader what to do. For example, a period means stop. Remember the old telegrams that used the word "stop" instead of periods? They sounded extremely funny when read aloud. We do not "read" our punctuation marks unless we are reading or dictating to someone who is taking down the information and needs to know the exact punctuation the reader prefers. Rather, punctuation serves as a silent system of signals and expression.

"Punctured Punctuation"

In *Feel Free to Write: A Guide for Business and Professional People,* author John Keenan mentions a customs clerk who was supposed to write: "All foreign fruit-plants are free from duty." But he wrote: "All foreign fruit, plants are free from duty." The error—one little comma—cost the United States government $2 million before the sentence could be changed.

Quick Rules for Correct Punctuation

1. A period goes at the end of a declarative sentence, e.g., Joshua fought the battle of Jericho.
2. Avoid run-on sentences by separating them and adding periods, e.g., "The client grabbed the crutches and ran down the corridor she fell before she reached the stairs." *Correct:* "The client grabbed the crutches and ran down the corridor. She fell before she reached the stairs."
3. Do not put a comma between the subject and verb of a sentence. *Incorrect:* "Inexperienced writers, may not know how to handle a difficult topic." *Correct:*

Inexperienced writers may not know how to handle a difficult topic."

4.   Do not use a comma between two separate, but related statements. Use a semicolon, e.g., *Incorrect:* "The chart was misplaced, it should have been hung on the patient's bed." *Correct:* "The chart was misplaced; it should have been hung on the patient's bed."

5.   Put commas between words in a series, e.g., "The office manager ordered paper, envelopes, paper clips, pencils, pens, and Krazy Glue." (Some styles, such as Associated Press style, prefer to leave out the comma after the next-to-last word in the series, e.g., "...pencils, pens and Krazy Glue.")

6.   Use commas to separate a person's name from his or her title in a sentence, e.g., "Dr. Bennett Rhodes, chairman of the chemistry department, gave a lecture." **But**, "Chemistry department chairman Dr. Bennett Rhodes gave a lecture."

7.   Use commas properly in quotations. *Incorrect:* "My client seems unwilling to cooperate with the rehab staff" Ms. Wilson said. *Correct:* "My client seems unwilling to cooperate with the rehab staff," Ms. Wilson said. *Incorrect:* "Go the whole nine yards," the therapist told his client. "And you'll be stronger for it." *Correct:* "Go the whole nine yards," the therapist told his client, "and you'll be stronger for it." *Incorrect:* "Yes my father will be here soon," Mary said. *Correct:* "Yes, my father will be here soon," Mary said.

8.   Use commas in appositions, e.g., "Mr. Macton, the nastiest weasel in America, cut our Christmas bonuses in half this year." "Allison, who rarely complained of pain, had a bad night." "My only cousin, Janice, lives in Delaware." (**But**, if I had more than one cousin: "My cousin Janice lives in Delaware.") "*The Encyclopedia of Vitamins, Minerals, and Supplements*, published in January 1996, is for professionals and lay people."

9. Use commas when two or more adjectives modify one noun, e.g., "Grandmother was a tiny, gentle, loving person."

10. Use a comma after an introductory clause or phrase, e.g., "When Jessica began to cook, her cat jumped off the refrigerator." (Think of the confusion that might occur if the comma were left out: We'd picture Jessica cooking her cat before we could adjust our thoughts.) If the introductory clause or phrase is very short, no comma is necessary, e.g., "For lunch the client ordered corned beef hash."

11. Use a comma between independent clauses joined by a conjunction, e.g., "Not every patient participates well in self-care, but I now have a patient who is highly motivated."

12. Use commas in parenthetical expressions, e.g., "The newborn weighed eight pounds, assuming the scale is correct." "Gravity, as far as we know, has been described but not explained."

13. Use a comma after a transitional phrase, e.g., "On the other hand, the nurse may have forgotten her keys and unwittingly caused confusion." "In fact, sweetgum trees are beautiful and popular." "Therefore, our teamwork has been a success."

14. Use commas in direct address, e.g., "Tell us, Mrs. Jones, what you believe is the problem." "Mary Ann, we all love you."

15. Use a comma after interrogative tags and mild interjections, e.g., "The OT was excellent, wasn't she?" "Well, there's no accounting for individual taste."

16. Use commas in dates, e.g., February 2, 1994. **But**, March 1996 or 10 March 1996 (no comma necessary).

17. Use commas in large numerals, e.g., "His yearly income was $3,765,000."

18. Use commas in addresses, e.g., "To contact the Editorial Director, write to SLACK Incorporated, 6900 Grove Road, Thorofare, NJ 08086."

19. Use a colon after the salutation in business letters, e.g., Dear Ms. Drummond: **But**, in a friendly letter, use a comma, e.g., Dear Johnny,

20. Use an apostrophe to form the possessive of singular nouns, e.g., the baby's toy, Mark's story, a reporter's question.

21. Use an apostrophe to form the possessive of plural nouns, e.g., bankers' hours, patients' rights, therapists' association. **But**, a name such as Sears is not a possessive form.

22. Use an apostrophe to form the possessive of a proper noun that ends in s, e.g., Kübler-Ross' book, Massachusetts' laws, Jones' estate. This can be done other ways, according to other styles, e.g., Kübler-Ross's book, James's car, etc.

23. **Do not** use an apostrophe to indicate a plural form, e.g., the Navarra's, the Burgess's, the Lundrigan's. *Correct:* the Navarras, the Burgesses, the Lundrigans.

24. **Do not** use an apostrophe if a word is already in the possessive form, e.g., yours, ours, his, hers, etc.

25. Use the dash—also known as an em-dash—as emphatic commas. An em-dash is a long dash; it equals three dashes together with no spaces between and no spaces before or after, e.g., How one spends his time—how long is a day?—mirrors how one wants to be remembered.

26. Use a hyphen to break a long word onto the next line, e.g., pro-crastination. Consult your dictionary for proper breaks.

27. Use a hyphen between two or more words that modify a noun, e.g., a hard-and-fast rule, three-foot lengths, laissez-faire attitude.

Author John Keenan quoted John Benbow, who wrote in the Oxford University Press style book, "If you take the hyphen seriously, you will surely go mad." My co-author Peggy Lundrigan, who with fiendish glee calls me the "Queen of Hyphens," leaves hyphens out deliberately so I can get my jollies putting them in.

Well, you now have the general idea of punctuation.
And that's all I've got to say about that.

Chapter 8
On Style

Write With a "Bite"

Writing is a lot like trying to bite your elbow; it may be a lot easier to bite someone else's elbow. In any case, good writing, stylish writing, ought to have a bite—your unique bite—to it. Writing without a bite tends either to be bland and forgettable, or a bark that amounts to nothing. That's the best way I know to get you started thinking about style.

Use a Style That Pleases

In his book *Feel Free to Write: A Guide for Business and Professional People*, John Keenan defines style as "The product of many choices the writer makes during the writing process. These choices are influenced not only by the writer's personality, but also by other limitations and concerns. The subject itself, the writer's role with respect to readers as he or she sees it, command of language, purpose—all affect style. Since style is both personal and complex, you might wonder whether anyone has the right to make value judgments, labeling one style 'good,' another 'bad.'

"If all writing were only self-expression, it would take a braver person than I am to sit in judgment. But the kind of writing we're discussing in this book is functional writing. It is written to analyze, inform, or persuade, and it is aimed at a specific audience. Therefore, the best style is one that pleases because it places the fewest obstacles between reader and writer. Like a pleasant stream, a readable style seems to carry the reader from one point to another, not to make him struggle upstream like a salmon."

Everything's in Style

Nearly everything we know possesses style in some way or other. Clothing, food, behavior, customs, ideas all bespeak a style. No style is incorrect. Think of styles in art: Cubism, Surrealism, Impressionism, Abstract Expressionism, etc. Which is wrong? None, of course. They are merely different from one another, each intending to express an individual point of view while containing some elements that are recognizably similar to a collective point of view.

Fred Astaire once said: "The higher up you go, the more mistakes you're allowed. Right at the top, if you make enough of them, it's considered to be your style."

Style Is What Makes Writing Distinctive

The minute you hear language to the effect of "To be, or not to be, that is the question," you can identify the author. A Cole Porter song lyric is easily recognized. When Tony Bennett starts his hallmark song, "I Left My Heart in San Francisco," you hear a unique style and voice. Good poetry has a distinctive voice; e.g., you can distinguish the language of Robert Frost from that of e.e. cummings. The one catch to developing style is not to imitate anyone else, but to stay in your own truth and tell your side of the story they way you naturally would tell it.

Designers of Literary Style

Just as there is no one correct way to paint or prepare green beans or put an outfit together, there is no one correct literary style. However, there are several styles that have been formulated to suit various types of writing.

Among the "designers" are the Univeristy of Chicago Press' *A Manual of Style*; Kate L. Turabian's *A Manual for Writers of Term Papers, Theses, and Dissertations*; *The New York Times Manual of Style and Usage*; the United Press International style, *The Associated Press Stylebook and Libel Manual;* Strunk and White's *The Elements of Style*; the Modern Language Association (MLA); American Psychological Association (APA) style; and guides put out by various publishers, including St. Martin's Press; Scott, Foresman; Prentice Hall; Merriam-Webster; and other publishers.

So Many Styles, So Little Time

Why are there so many styles when one might fit all? Although excess seems to be the great American vice, I think it would be a dull world without variety; in fact, the world is a field of all possibilities.

In addition, having several styles to choose from helps people who are not professional writers create an ordered, presentable research paper or thesis and encourages consistency of spelling, punctuation, and word usage.

Love Me, Love My Style

When I was an undergraduate, I discovered that each professor preferred a specific style and instructed students to use it for research papers. So, if a professor favored MLA, I used my own style, and if she dictated the use of Chicago, I used my own style. Most of the time (with the exception of my thesis) I did as I pleased, which I thought was fine as long as I gave all the required information and proved consistent in format.

Of course, I majored in art, the "anything goes" department, so I do not recommend your doing this in undergraduate and graduate health programs. But I must tell you that never has any teacher, including in a graduate program, objected to my research-paper style. For example, I have always used the same format for a bibliography not to be a maverick, but because I believe it is the most accessible format for the reader: Bradbury, Ray, *Zen in the Art of Writing*, Bantam Books, New York, 1990.

To my knowledge, it does not adhere to any designated style, but it's clean and simple. Using commas between each component—author, title, publisher, place, and year— is easier to remember than periods, colons, parentheses, and other punctuation. But if you're under the gun to use a particular style, I forgive you. At any rate, using a specific style is not terribly difficult. In fact, it is supposed to make writing a lot easier, something like following a cooking recipe, except you dream up your own ingredients.

Turabian and Chicago: Bradbury, Ray. *Zen in the Art of Writing.* New York: Bantam Books, 1990.

APA: Bradbury, R. (1990). *Zen in the Art of Writing.* New York. Bantam Books.

Council of Biology Editors (CBE): Bradbury, R. *Zen in the Art of Writing.* New York: Bantam Books, 1990.

Bibliography or Hieroglyphics?

Just try reading the bibliography of some medical or other technical books. Invariably it will contain mysterious abbreviations, strange punctuation, and other quirky characteristics, and it will be in small, fine, dense print so you become bleary-eyed after a minute or two. For example, "Mieszala P. Postburn psychological adaptation: An overview. *CCQ* 1978 Dec; 1(3):93-111" is crammed into the bibliography of *The Lippincott Manual of Nursing Practice (3rd ed.)*, 1982. I'd have to call a reference librarian to find out what *CCQ* is, and 1(3):93-111 I presume refers to volume number and pages, but I'd have to look it up as well.

I came across other bibliographical entries of the nearly baffling kind in the American Medical Association's "*Code of Medical Ethics (1994 edition)*: Boozang, Death Wish: Resuscitating Self-Determination for the Critically Ill, 35 Ariz. L. Rev. 23, 23, 28, 52 (1993) [2.22, 8.08]" and "Daar, A Clash at the Bedside: Patient Autonomy v. A Physician's Professional Conscience, 44 Hastings L.J. 1241, 1257, 1268, 1286 (1993)[2.20, 2.22]."

If you are familiar with the abbreviations and numbers, bravo. But others may not read these entries with ease. And to boot, no first names appear for the authors. What if there are 17 different Boozangs writing articles on death wishes? Too bad we can't purchase an official secret decoder ring for snags like this.

Strunk Style Tenets

The late Cornell University Professor William Strunk, Jr. set forth rules of style that include such bold instructions as:

1.   Place yourself in the background.
2.   Write in a way that comes naturally.
3.   Work from a suitable design.
4.   Write with nouns and verbs.
5.   Revise and rewrite.
6.   Do not overwrite.
7.   Do not overstate.
8.   Avoid the use of qualifiers.
9.   Do not affect a breezy manner.
10.   Use orthodox spelling.
11.   Do not explain too much.
12.   Do not construct awkward adverbs.
13.   Make sure the reader knows who is speaking.
14.   Avoid fancy words.
15.   Do not use dialect unless your ear is good.
16.   Be clear.
17.   Do not inject opinion.
18.   Use figures of speech sparingly.
19.   Do not take shortcuts at the cost of clarity.
20.   Avoid foreign languages.
21.   Prefer the standard to the offbeat.

Strunk and White's *The Elements of Style* has long been revered, but I don't think a writer absolutely must choose one style ethic and stick to it forever. Writers like to play with words. E.B. White wrote, "Style takes its final shape more from attitudes of mind than from principles of composition, for as an elderly practitioner once remarked, 'Writing is an act of faith, not a trick of grammar.' This moral observation would have no place in a rulebook were it not that style is the writer, and therefore what a man is, rather than what he knows, will at last determine his style."

Style Also Refers to Expressions, Points of Grammar, and Punctuation

A Manual of Style prefers a date to be written without punctuation, e.g., 20 November 1995, or May 1996. An older style requires commas, e.g., November 20, 1995 or May, 1996.

Notice, too, that after an expression such as i.e. (meaning that is) or e.g. (meaning for example), use a comma. See the sentence above.

Find a Style Bible and Get "Religion"

If you are not planning to hang up your stethoscope or turn in your motor-coordination equipment to strike out as a writer, your best bet is to purchase a good, new book on a style that appeals to you or that is most frequently used in your field. Learn that style inside out. Think of the style book as your tool box, in which may be found a hammer, screwdriver, crowbar, pliers, wrench, and other gadgets you know precisely how to use for various repairs. Refer to the book often when you are writing a paper, article, or other piece. *The New York Times*' review of Strunk and White's style book, which is ever loyal to plain English style, included the statement: "Buy it, study it, enjoy it. It's as timeless as a book can be in our age of volubility."

Do Your Best to Include Stylish Details

In her book *Bird by Bird: Some Instructions on Writing and Life*, Anne Lamott wrote: "Write down everything you can remember about every birthday or Christmas or Seder or Easter or whatever, every relative who was there. Write down all the stuff you swore you'd never tell another soul....Scratch around for details: what people ate, listened to, wore—those terrible petaled swim caps, the men's awful trunks, the cocktail dress your voluptuous aunt wore that was so slinky she practically needed the Jaws of Life to get out of it...Describe the trench coats and stoles and car coats, what they revealed and what they covered up...Remember that you own what happened to you."

If you heed Lamott's call for details, they can make all the difference and allow the emergence of your style: the odd things you notice, the ironies, the way you describe a facial expression or a patient's posture in a hospital bed, the way you prepare a reader's psyche to feel the joy of a 20-year-old client with a head injury at being able to apply mascara successfully during an OT session. The possibilities for description and details are endless, and they are you, the writer.

Style Is Your Own "Voice"

Lamott also wrote: "Your anger and damage and grief are a way to the truth. We don't have much truth to express unless we have gone into those rooms and closets and woods and abysses that we were told not to go in to. When we have gone and looked around for a while, just breathing and taking it in—then we will be able to speak in our own voice and to stay in the present moment. And that moment is home."

Style and Publication

Although I've never heard anything but praise for Strunk and White, publishers and editors feel free to change whatever style you use to the style their publications prefer. *The New York Times*, for example, developed its own manual of style and usage.

In one article I did for the *Times*, I used the phrase "according to the *Encyclopaedia Britannica*," which was done routinely at the *Asbury Park Press*. The *Times* editor told me, "We don't use 'according to.'" She changed it to "The *Encyclopaedia Britannica* says...." Personally, I never dreamed those heavy volumes could talk, but, as songwriter Paul Simon puts it, who am I to blow against the wind?

Chapter 9
On Tone

Written Tone Imitates Spoken Tone

You know when a person says something sarcastically, or sympathetically, sweetly, angrily, arrogantly, or distractedly. Tone is simply the tone of voice you use either speaking or writing. Remember your mother's crescendo as she said when you were a bratty child, "I'm going to count to three..."? Her tone was threatening. A person cooing to a baby uses a non-threatening, often high-pitched, smiley tone of voice. Lovers speak softly and sensually to each other, hence, a soft, sensual, intimate tone.

Name That Tone

Read what you write aloud to yourself so you pick up on the tone of voice you've chosen. If you are writing a memo to your supervisor, be careful your tone is not that of a scolded puppy or Attila the Hun. Write honestly, but don't become tone-deaf. On the other hand, if you are writing a rebuttal to a debate question, your tone can be as bellicose as you wish, provided such bellicosity is an acceptable aspect of the forensics in which you are engaged.

Tone Is Emotional

John Keenan writes that we should be sensitive to words. The choice of one word over another may make all the difference in how the reader perceives the meaning and emotion of a phrase or sentence. "Advertising and public relations writers are careful with connotations (emotional associations attached to words)," Keenan wrote. "They know nobody wants to live in an alley, but if the street is called a court it becomes more attractive, even though it is not any wider from curb to curb."

He goes on to explain that physicians, particularly those who do not read good literature, and other professionals who tend not to read any literature outside of their fields, often have a tin ear when it comes to words and the tone of their writing. They may overuse the passive voice and rely on stereotyped sentence structure and hackneyed beginnings. In sum, their writing comes across as impersonal and perhaps haughty.

Read to Improve Your Sense of Tone

Most writing gurus recommend that health professionals break away as often as possible from professional literature. Read a classic novel. Read poetry. Read the editorial and Op-Ed pages of the nation's top newspapers. Read good quality best-sellers. In his essay, "The Writer as Student and Teacher," in a Bread Loaf anthology entitled *Writers on Writing*, David Huddle writes, "Within their individual sensibilities—the true source of originality—writers carry around what they've learned from other writers."

From Ellen Bryant Voigt's "On Tone," *Writers on Writing*, here is more information on tone: "Most of us can identify tone in life—and depend on it for meaning. When you're in bed, at the verge of sleep, and you hear voices in the next apartment, what you register is tone. The actual words don't pass through the wall, but from the volume, pitch, relative stress, pacing, and rhythmic pattern of the speech you reconstruct the emotional content of the conversation. It's what the dog registers when you talk to him sternly or playfully—the form of the emotion behind or within the words. It's also what can allow an obscenity to pass for an endearment, or a term of affection to become suddenly an insult."

Chapter 10
On Paraphrasing, Plagiarism, Deadlines, Writer's Block, and Ghostwriting

Paraphrasing, or Restating Someone Else's Words

First, as in health care, do no harm. In other words, maintain the original meaning of the sentences you paraphrase. If you do not understand what is written, or if you think you understand but you're haunted by doubt, quote directly and credit your source. If you choose to paraphrase, be certain your version of the text does not alter the original author's meaning.

Do not take a simple phrase and make it a difficult one for the sake of paraphrasing. Making difficult writing simpler and more accessible to your reader, however, is fine. Dense, overly technical or awkward language should be paraphrased. You must credit your source even if you change the words.

Understand Plagiarism

Webster's Collegiate Dictionary defines plagiarism as "to steal or pass off (the ideas or words of another) as one's own; to use (a created production) without crediting the source; to commit literary theft."

My best and unflagging advice on plagiarizing is DON'T. Pilfering someone else's writing, i.e., passing it off as your own, not giving credit to the original author, is despicable. It could lead to a nasty lawsuit, the loss of a job, and personal humiliation. Plagiarists: Go directly to jail; do not collect $200. Moreover, anyone who feels the need to plagiarize is not a writer; he or she is a thief.

Understand What Deadline Means

A deadline is a date (and perhaps even a time of day) when an article, chapter, book, or term paper is due to be handed in to either an instructor, professor, or publisher.

Meet deadlines on time or ahead of time. Only the most genuinely hideous excuse may—and I say may— be considered.

Learn to budget your writing time. No editor wants to hear about your son's appendectomy or your niece's bat mitzvah that prevented you from finishing an article. Editors have carpenter ants in their pants. They hate to wait and often will not wait for you to deliver your piece. Consequently, you may not be invited to write anything else for that publication. Deadlines are set for a reason. Editors need editing time, and production people need production time. It's teamwork, really, so pull your weight.

I must recount this story, however. A student (a grown man with a family of his own) in a master's-level course told the professor he needed some more time to complete the term paper required because he was fired suddenly from his job, his wife left home and filed for divorce, his father died, and one of his children was hospitalized with pneumonia all at the same time. As preposterous as it sounds, the man was telling the professor the truth. Said the professor coolly: "So?"

Just remember that grim tale when your deadline comes around. Because you may encounter the same inhuman detachment, make sure you foresee as well as possible how to get your assignment in on time.

Writer's Block

"Phooey on writer's block. It's a myth," I've heard many people say. Most people associate writer's block with a lack of ideas on what to write. But I tend to believe it's resistance (which often involves complicated emotional issues), plain old procrastination, or an intriguing euphemism for depression, which does indeed interfere with writing and many other types of work and functioning. I tend to suffer "depression blocks" because I have too many ideas swirling like Dante's *Inferno* in my head, and all that action has the power to paralyze me for a while. What do I do? I take to my bed and give myself permission not to do anything at the moment. I eat Peanut Chews as though I were Mr. Goldenberg's personal advocate. And I make lists of teensy-weensy tasks and cross them off one by one as I complete them. One teensy-weensy task I perform when I feel "brain dead" is wrapping Christmas gifts. It's mindless but useful. After I wrap about 20, I'm usually ready to go back to my manuscript.

Those of you who experience true "writer's block" as a result of feeling overwhelmed or bereft of ideas and approaches to an assignment may need to talk to a peer counselor, a guidance counselor or advisor, a psychologist, or other writers who are willing to share their horror stories so you don't feel alone with the problem.

There is also this theory espoused by many writers and teachers: If a project seems too foreign, too difficult, too much for you, then it probably is. Regroup and alter the piece of writing to suit your ability, your present mindset, and your general lifestyle and day-to-day responsibilities.

Rehearsing

One editor said when he saw writers wandering about the newsroom, schmoozing, staring into space, doodling, or somehow looking as though they weren't doing what the company pays them for, they were rehearsing. Writers do this. They seem to be doing something else, but actually they're mentally preparing to write a piece. It's a mini-block, I suppose, that is easily overcome. I rehearse when I do the dishes, stand in the yard waiting for my puppy to finish his business, watch television, meditate, or gab on the phone. In fact, I spend half my life rehearsing (asleep or awake), and the other half writing.

What to Do if You're "Blocked"

If depression blocks are short-lived, take heart and work like a house afire between them. If you find you can't work day after day for long periods of time, the diagnosis may not be a simple dry spell, but something more serious. **Get professional help.**

However, if you swear you're not depressed, it's just that nothing good seems to be flowing at the moment, go to a movie (the right movie can have a powerful motivating effect), take a karate lesson, have a beer, drive to the reservoir for a short hike, buy yourself a present at Lord & Taylor's—do anything that helps you feel free, light, and clearheaded.

Then go back to the typewriter or computer and type nonsense words, free associations, or whatever comes to mind about your topic. Most of the time, the "garbage" will eventually turn into prose. Be patient. Have faith. Remember, if you can talk about your topic, you can write about it.

What Is Ghostwriting?

The best advice on ghostwriting I've come across is from Scott Edelstein's book, *The Writer's Book of Checklists*. Here I will condense Edelstein's 10 tips on ghostwriting.

1.   Ghostwriting means a) you write the piece and someone else gets credit as author; b) you write something in collaboration with someone else, but you receive no by-line; c) you do most of the writing, but you share a by-line with another; or d) you write a piece under a pseudonym.
2.   Publishers, writers, literary agents, celebrities, and government officials often hire ghostwriters.
3.   Sign a written agreement, preferably one you write yourself, in advance.
4.   Ghostwriting contracts are negotiable.
5.   Payment for ghostwriting may be a flat fee, an hourly fee, a percentage of sales, or an initial fee plus a percentage of sales.

6.   Never agree to ghostwrite on spec—to be paid only if the piece sells.
7.   Ghostwriters typically earn $25 to $60 an hour plus royalties.
8.   Be wary of working with eccentric, unstable, unavailable, absurdly busy people, or anyone who makes the job impossible.
9.   It's tough to acquire ghostwriting assignments, but offer your services to book packagers, agents, book publishers who have published your work, and editorial services.
10. If you have a gut feeling that the project isn't going to work, back out as gracefully as you can.

To Scott Edelstein's astute advice I add this from my own rotten experiences: Be extremely cautious about doing a biography of a person who is alive. I wrote two biographical books about artists. They caused me so much aggravation that I contemplated murdering my subjects and then, while serving a life sentence, making up hideous things to write about them. About 10 years ago, an editor at Rutgers University Press told me they wouldn't even consider publishing a book on a living artist. I wonder if their policy has changed, and, if it has, may the Force be with those poor authors.

Chapter 11
On Editing, Proofreading, and Encouraging Your Colleagues

Pain in the Editing

Author Marcia Lerner says editing, a painful process, is the main work of writing, but the results are worth it. Let's think of editing not as painful, but rather as an incredibly delicate operation performed under anesthesia. All manner of horrific things can be done when a patient is under anesthesia, but those horrific things, wrought of highly skilled surgeons' and nurses' hands, often mean life or death to the patient. Surgeons know exactly what and where and how to cut; they excise only the undesirable parts so the healthy parts continue to thrive. This, dear readers, is editing.

Bad Haircuts vs. Good Editing

Novice writers tend to fall madly in love with their words and can't bear watching them hit the editorial-office floor. To be certain, there are lousy editors who simply chop here and there, as though giving a bad haircut. These are the ones who tend not to be knowledgeable or interested in the subject matter. But more often than not, editors are good at identifying and excising the chaff and preserving the best of a piece. *Chicago Tribune* writer Michael A. Lev had some funny and painful things to say about editors and editing:

"The relationship between writer and editor has many foundations: There is trust, respect, and artistic vision. But at the core, one finds the ugly truth: fear, skepticism, and disdain.

"It's an unavoidable fact because editors by definition are critics and meddlers. They exist because the process of writing is built on the premise that the writer, unlike the painter, shouldn't—or can't—do the job right alone. Chefs don't have editors. Neither do accountants."

Lev said even Thomas Jefferson's *Declaration of Independence* was heavily edited. "It's got scribbled-out words, along with blacked-out paragraphs and numerous rewritten phrases inserted by the document's chief editor, Benjamin Franklin," Lev wrote.

For example, Jefferson's original copy cited "these truths to be sacred and undeniable." Franklin changed "sacred and undeniable" to "self-evident." Biographers say although Jefferson pouted a great deal over the changes, they did in fact improve the work.

What Infection Where?

I remember writing a grant-proposal anecdote about a 19-year-old woman who, said a visiting nurse, was sitting on the couch, sucking her thumb, as her four little children cried or picked at their scabied skin. The toddler had an infected penis. I thought the whole picture would have looked so grim to a funder that he'd whip out his checkbook on reading that sentence alone. But my supervisor changed the penile infection to an ear infection. I say write the truth. Why soften such a horrid story, especially in a grant proposal?

Of all the editors I have ever worked with, this supervisor was the pits—not an editor at all. I always say a really good editor makes my writing better, which makes me look good, and I always say a good editor is hard to find.

Major Editorial Questions to Ask Yourself

You may have to write a rough draft (which, says Anne Lamott with a grittier word, may be scatological in nature) and edit it several times. Each time, your eye should be more critical and merciless than the last time. Merciless, I repeat. Don't treat yourself to praise and retention the way you'd coo over a child's kindergarten drawing. (Would anyone actually tell a child she should have redone the yellow part and made the lines heavier?) Think of the surgery—life or death, diseased vs. healthy. Now go back to your piece and pretend you're the surgeon. A surgeon has no mercy for the disease. Neither does the patient. Ask yourself the following questions as you edit:

1. Does the lead put its arms around me and draw me to it? How can I change it so it is concise but powerful?
2. Is the piece logically arranged? Do I go easily from one important point to another? Do I digress and thus detract from the piece with a lot of trivial stuff?
3. If I were a lay reader, would I know what I am talking about?
4. Is my tone correct, or is it too terse, too soft, too dry, etc.?
5. Do I really really really need this word or that phrase? If the answer is no, get rid of it. No sticky fingers allowed.
6. Are my verb tenses and point of view consistent?
7. Does each sentence say precisely what I mean?
8. Is my writing honest? Is it me or some phony? Have I written the truth and done it well?
9. How's my grammar? Did I goof on usage or punctuation?
10. Is my voice active rather than passive?
11. Do I unnecessarily use jargon, technical words, unacceptable words?
12. Did I use clichés and hackneyed words?
13. Have I described people and things adequately, or have I over-described them to make my copy dense and difficult?
14. Did I end the piece well?
15. Am I pleased enough with the piece after editing thoroughly to proofread it?

The Proof(reading) Is in the Pudding

Proofreading has but one commandment: **nit-pick like crazy**. Find every typo, every incorrect comma, colon, period, hyphen, and apostrophe, every lower-case letter that should be upper-case. Common typos are those that require transposition of letters, such as form instead of from, and misspellings, such as pubic instead of public.

When a writer proofreads using a word processor or computer, it is possible to overlook words that had been changed or should be eliminated. Too often they remain in the text in addition to editorial changes. Spellcheck functions may also be unable to detect words that should be cut because all spellcheck does is allow words that are not misspelled to stay in the text.

Bad breaks at the end of sentences (this occurs in typeset copy or galleys) should be corrected, such as congressio-nal. Hunt for words that should be capitalized and are not.

Peck for semi-colons that should be colons. See that underlining or italicization are correct. Separate words that unwittingly got stuck together. Check again for consistent usage of language and style.

When I was a reporter, the editorial-page editor daily asked me to proofread the editorial pages before they went to press. I found all sorts of mistakes even after three other editors read the copy. I knew then I was a very sick woman—I was determined to be the best proofreader in the universe.

Nonetheless, I encourage you to let other eyes fall upon your copy after you've seen it so many times you don't know what's there or not. You never know what another's eye will find—and perhaps save you some embarrassment.

Encouraging Your Colleagues

Please do. We are all in this health care whirl together, and we need everyone's point of view to help us evolve. As I finish this book, I hope I have encouraged the writer in you to come out of the locker room and show us your yellow polka-dot bikini. (Remember that silly song?) Teach us what you know. Describe what you've felt and experienced. Explain ideas we might not understand if not for your ability to make them painlessly accessible and memorable. I admit writing full-time makes for a crazed, roller-coaster life, but if you decide to write either

occasionally or frequently, I assure you it will reap some
fine rewards. Let me know what happens.

Epilogue

"You've seen them everywhere: chatterbox children who become tongue-tied on paper; talkative teenagers who monopolize the telephone, but insist they can't write...I spent 3 years and traveled 22,000 miles across the United States, and I believe that today's students are at risk. The danger lies in their becoming part of the 'I hate to write' generation, sons and daughters of 'I hate to write' parents."—Arlene Silberman, *Growing Up Writing*

Like Ms. Silberman, I believe we can change "I hate to write" to "I have to write because I have something valuable to say."

Bibliography

Alley, Michael, *The Craft of Scientific Writing*, Prentice-Hall, Inc., Englewood Cliffs, NJ, 1987.

American Medical Association "News Release," Chicago, October 4, 1995.

Angione, Howard, ed., *The Associated Press Stylebook and Libel Manual*, The Associated Press, New York, 1977.

Asbury Park Press Editorial Handbook, Asbury Park Press, Neptune, NJ.

Axelrod, Rise B., and Cooper, Charles R., *The St. Martin's Guide to Writing*, St. Martin's Press, New York, 1991.

Barzun, Jacques, *Simple & Direct: A Rhetoric for Writers*, Harper & Row Publishers, New York, 1975.

Beebe, Linda, ed., *Professional Writing for the Human Services*, National Association of Social Workers, Washington, DC, 1993.

Bennett, William J., *The Book of Virtues: A Treasury of Great Moral Stories*, Simon & Schuster, New York, 1993.

Bernhard, Elizabeth A., Feder, Jody, and Lin, Alvin C., eds., *1997 Guide to Federal Funding for Governments and Non-Profits*, Government Information Services, Arlington, VA, Vols. 1 & 2, 1997.

Brande, Dorothea, *Becoming a Writer*, Jeremy P. Tarcher, Inc., Los Angeles, 1981.

Brooks, Terri, *Words' Worth: A Handbook on Writing and Selling Nonfiction*, St. Martin's Press, New York, 1989.

Burnham, Sophy, *For Writers Only*, Ballantine Books, New York, 1994.

Cappon, Rene J., *The Word: An Associated Press Guide to Good News Writing*, The Associated Press, New York, 1982.

Carroll, Lewis, *The Annotated Alice,* Branshall House, Clarkson N. Potter, Inc., New York, 1960.

Cheney, Theodore A. Rees, *Writing Creative Nonfiction*, Ten Speed Press, Berkeley, CA, 1991.

Cox, Don Richard, and Giddens, Elizabeth, *Crafting Prose*, Harcourt Brace Jovanovich Publishers, New York, 1991.

Dickens, Charles, *Hard Times*, Bantam Books, New York, 1981 ed.

Dillard, Annie, *The Writing Life*, Harper & Row Publishers, New York, 1989.

Dion, Susan, *Write Now: Maintaining a Creative Spirit While Homebound and Ill*, Puffin Foundation, Ltd., Teaneck, NJ, 1994.

DiTillio, Lawrence G., "A Solid Sense of Structure," *Writer's Digest*, February, 1997, p. 19.

Dyer, Wayne W., *You'll See It When You Believe It*, Avon Books, New York, 1989.

Edelstein, Scott, *The Writer's Book of Checklists*, Writer's Digest Books, Cincinnati, OH, 1991.

Elbow, Peter, *Writing Without Teachers*, Oxford University Press, New York, 1973.

Estell, Kenneth, and Wisner-Broyles, Lana, eds., *Corporate Giving Directory, 19th ed.*, The Taft Group, New York, 1998.

Fedler, Fred, *Reporting for the Print Media (3rd ed.)*, Harcourt Brace Jovanovich Publishers, New York, 1973.

Goethe, Johann Wolfgang von, *The Sorrows of Young Werther*, New American Library, New York, 1962 ed.

Goldberg, Natalie, *Writing Down the Bones*, Shambhala Publishing Inc., Boston, 1986.

Hacker, Diana, *The Bedford Handbook for Writers*, Bedford Books, St. Martin's Press, Boston, 1991.

Hairston, Maxine, and Ruszkiewicz, John J., *The Scott Foresman Handbook for Writers (2nd ed.)*, HarperCollins Publishers, New York, 1991.

Hall, Donald, and Emblen, D.L., *A Writer's Reader*, HarperCollins Publishers, New York, 1991.

Harman, Willis, and Rheingold, Howard, *Higher Creativity: Liberating the Unconscious for Breakthrough Insights*, Jeremy P. Tarcher, Inc., New York, 1984.

Hughes, Riley, *How to Write Creatively*, Franklin Watts, New York, 1980.

Hulme, Kathryn, *The Nun's Story*, Little, Brown and Company, Boston, 1956.

Iacocca, Lee, *Talking Straight*, Bantam Books, New York, 1989.

Jordan, Lewis, ed., *The New York Times Manual of Style and Usage*, Times Books, New York, 1976.

Keenan, John, *Feel Free to Write: A Guide for Business and Professional People*, John Wiley & Sons, New York, 1982.

Kilpatrick, James J., *The Writer's Art*, Andrews, McMeel & Parker Inc., New York, 1984.

Kirszner, Laurie G., and Mandell, Stephen R., *Patterns for College Writing: A Rhetorical Reader and Guide*, St. Martin's Press, New York, 1986.

Kübler-Ross, Elisabeth, *On Death and Dying*, MacMillan Publishing Co., New York, 1969.

Lamm, Kathryn, *10,000 Ideas for Term Papers, Projects, Reports & Speeches*, MacMillan Publishing Company, Inc., New York, 1995.

Lamott, Anne, *Bird by Bird: Some Instructions on Writing and Life*, Anchor Books, Doubleday, New York, 1994.

Leavitt, Hart Day, and Sohn, David A., *Look, Think & Write: Using pictures to stimulate thinking and improve your writing*, National Textbook Company, Lincolnwood, IL, 1985.

Lerner, Marcia, *The Princeton Review Writing Smart*, Villard Books, New York, 1994.

Lev, Michael A., "We hold these truths to be sacred and undeniable...," *Asbury Park Press*, July 5, 1995, p. A9.

Mahony, Patrick J., *Freud as a Writer*, Yale University Press, New Haven, CT, 1987.

A Manual of Style, The University of Chicago Press, Chicago, IL, 1969.

Marano, Hara Estroff, "We Met at the Office...," *Psychology Today*, March/April 1995.

McCuen, Jo Ray, and Winkler, Anthony C., *Rewriting Writing: A Rhetoric and Reader*, Harcourt Brace Jovanovich Publishers, New York, 1990.

McLean, Rebecca, and McLeod, Denise, eds., *The Foundation Grants Index 1997*, The Foundation Center, USA, 1997.

McWilliams, Peter, *DO IT! Let's Get Off Our Buts*, Prelude Press, Los Angeles, 1994.

Means, Beth, and Lindner, Lindy, *Everything You Needed to Learn about Writing in High School But a) you were in love b) you have forgotten c) you fell asleep d) they didn't tell you e) all of the above*, Libraries Unlimited, Inc., Englewood, CO, 1989.

The Merriam-Webster Concise Handbook for Writers, Merriam-Webster Inc., Publishers, Springfield, MA, 1991.

Merriam-Webster's Collegiate Dictionary, 10th ed., Merriam-Webster Inc., Publishers, Springfield, MA, 1993.

Michener, James A., *The Novel,* Fawcett Crest Book, Ballantine Books, New York, 1991.

Miller, Robert K., *The Informed Argument: A Multidisciplinary Reader and Guide*, Harcourt Brace Jovanovich Publishers, New York, 1986.

Miller, Susan, *The Written World: Reading and Writing in Social Contexts*, Harper & Row Publishers, New York, 1989.

Mitchell, Margaret, *Gone With the Wind*, Macmillan and Co., New York, 1936.

Nightingale, Florence, *Notes on Nursing: What it is and what it is not*, Harrison and Sons, England, 1860.

O'Connor, Andrea B., *Writing for Nursing Publications*, SLACK Incorporated, Thorofare, NJ, 1988.

Otfinoski, Steve, *Putting It In Writing*, Scholastic Inc., New York, 1993.

Pack, Robert, and Parini, Jay, *Writers on Writing*, Middlebury College Press, University Press of New England, Hanover, NH, 1991.

Packer, Nancy Huddleston, and Timpane, John, *Writing Worth Reading: A Practical Guide*, St. Martin's Press, New York, 1986.

Panus, Jerrold, *Official Fundraising Almanac*, Pluribus Press, Inc., Chicago, IL, 1989.

Plotnik, Arthur, *The Elements of Editing: A Modern Guide for Editors and Journalists*, Collier Books, Macmillan Publishing Company, New York, 1982.

Prather, Hugh, *Notes to Myself: My Struggle to Become a Person*, Bantam Books, New York, 1981.

Prentice-Hall Author's Guide, Prentice-Hall, Inc., Englewood Cliffs, NJ, 1975.

Provost, Gary, *100 Ways to Improve Your Writing*, Mentor Books, Penguin Books USA Inc., New York, 1985.

Reinking, James A., and Hart, Andrew W., *Strategies for Successful Writing*, Prentice-Hall, Englewood Cliffs, NJ, 1986.

Rubins, Diane Teitel, *Scholastic's A+ Guide to Good Writing*, Scholastic, Inc., New York, 1980.

Safire, William, "Four-Letter Words," *The New York Times Magazine*, April 30, 1995.

Shaw, Fran Weber, *50 Ways to Help You Write*, Longmeadow Press, Stamford, CT, 1995.

Shipley, Joseph T., *In Praise of English: The Growth & Use of Language*, Times Books, New York, 1977.

Silberman, Arlene, *Growing Up Writing*, Random House, Inc., New York, 1989.

Skwire, David, *Writing with a Thesis: A Rhetoric and Reader*, Holt, Rinehart and Winston, New York, 1979.

Spence, Gerry, *How to Argue and Win Every Time*, St. Martin's Press, New York, 1996.

Spikol, Art, "Looking for Leads in All the Wrong Phrases?," *Writer's Digest*, January 1991, pp. 66-70.

Stonecipher, Harry W., *Editorial and Persuasive Writing: Opinion Functions of the News Media*, Communication Arts Books, Hastings House, Mamaroneck, New York, 1990.

Strunk, William, Jr., and White, E.B., *The Elements of Style*, The Macmillan Company, New York, 1962.

Trimmer, Joseph F., *Writing with a Purpose (10th ed.)*, Houghton Mifflin Company, Boston, 1992.

Turabian, Kate L., *A Manual for Writers of Term Papers, Theses, and Dissertations*, The University of Chicago Press, Chicago, 1973.

Turabian, Kate L., *Student's Guide for Writing College Papers*, The University of Chicago Press, Chicago, 1976.

Tyner, Thomas E., *Writing Voyage: An Integrated Process Approach to Basic Writing*, Wadsworth Publishing Company, Belmont, CA, 1988.

Ueland, Brenda, *If You Want To Write*, Graywolf Press, St. Paul, MN, 1987.

United Press International UPI Stylebook: The Authoritative Handbook for Writers, Editors & News Directors, National Textbook Company, Lincolnwood, IL, 1992.

Weiss, Edmond H., *The Writing System for Engineers and Scientists*, Prentice-Hall, Inc., Englewood Cliffs, NJ, 1982.

Williams, Joseph M., *Style: Toward Clarity and Grace*, The University of Chicago Press, Chicago, 1990.

Zinsser, William, *On Writing Well: An Informal Guide to Writing Nonfiction*, Harper Perennial, New York, 1990.

Index

*F*or your information

This book and many others on numerous different topics are available from SLACK Incorporated. For further information or a copy of our latest catalog, contact us at:

Professional Book Division
SLACK Incorporated
6900 Grove Road
Thorofare, NJ 08086 USA
Telephone: 1-609-848-1000
1-800-257-8290
Fax: 1-609-853-5991
E-mail: orders@slackinc.com
WWW: http://www.slackinc.com

We accept most major credit cards and checks or money orders in US dollars drawn on a US bank. Most orders are shipped within 72 hours.

Contact us for information on recent releases, forthcoming titles, and bestsellers. If you have a comment about this title or see a need for a new book, direct your correspondence to the Editorial Director at the above address.

*If you are an instructor, we can be reached at the address listed above or on the Internet at **educomps@slackinc.com** for specific needs.*

Thank you for your interest and we hope you found this work beneficial.